550 + Herbal Remedies and Natural Healing Techniques Inspired by Barbara O'Neill

A mind-opening book.

By Roberta Lane

TABLE OF CONTENTS

HYDRATION AND ELECTROLYTE BALANCE

Infusion of Herbal Electrolyte

Intended Use: Supports hydration and electrolyte balance with a blend of herbs known for their mineral content.

Ingredients:

- 1 tsp dried nettle leaf
- 1 tsp dried dandelion leaf
- 1 tsp dried hibiscus flowers
- 4 cups boiling water

Preparation:

1. Place the nettle leaf, dandelion leaf, and hibiscus flowers in a large teapot or jar.
2. Pour boiling water over the herbs and cover.
3. Allow to steep for 4-6 hours or overnight for a strong infusion.
4. Strain the liquid and refrigerate until cool.

How to Use: Consume 1-2 cups daily to ensure adequate hydration and replenishment of essential minerals.

Avocado and Spinach Blend

Intended Use: provides vital fats and nutrients for long-term energy and hydration.

Ingredients:

- 1 ripe avocado
- 2 cups fresh spinach
- 1 banana
- 2 cups coconut water
- Ice cubes (optional)

Preparation:

1. Combine avocado, spinach, banana, and coconut water in a blender.
2. Add ice cubes for a colder smoothie if preferred.
3. Blend until smooth and creamy.

4. Serve immediately.

How to Use: Drink this to hydrate and feed your body in the morning or as a post-workout snack.

Herbal Infusion Hydration Tea

Intended Use: combines a combination of hydrating herbs to support general hydration and restore minerals..

Ingredients:

- 1 tsp dried nettle leaf
- 1 tsp dried alfalfa leaf
- 1 tsp dried raspberry leaf
- 4 cups boiling water

Preparation:

1. Combine nettle, alfalfa, and raspberry leaf in a large teapot or heat-proof jar.
2. Pour boiling water over the herbs.
3. Cover and steep for 15-20 minutes.
4. Strain and serve the tea warm or chilled.

How to Use: To maintain hydrated, drink one to two cups each day, particularly in warmer weather or during times when you're exercising more.

Watermelon and Basil Refresher

Intended Use: Hydrates the body while providing essential vitamins and antioxidants.

Ingredients:

- 4 cups cubed watermelon
- A handful of fresh basil leaves
- Juice of ½ lemon

Preparation:

1. Blend watermelon cubes, basil leaves, and lemon juice until smooth.
2. Strain the mixture through a fine mesh sieve to remove any solids.
3. Serve the juice chilled for a refreshing hydration boost.

How to Use: On hot days or after exercise, sip on a glass of watermelon basil juice to immediately replenish your fluids.

Salty Electrolyte Drink with Lemonade

Intended Use: provides a homemade energy and hydration substitute for store-bought electrolyte drinks.

Ingredients:

- 4 cups filtered water
- Juice of 2 lemons
- ½ tsp Himalayan pink salt
- 2 tbsp honey or maple syrup

Preparation:

1. In a pitcher, combine water and fresh lemon juice.
2. Add Himalayan pink salt and honey or maple syrup, stirring until dissolved.
3. Adjust sweetness or saltiness to taste.

How to Use: Drink throughout the day to replace lost electrolytes and fluids, or after perspiring.

Mint Cucumber Refresher

Intended Use: has a mild detoxifying impact while cooling and hydrating the body.

Ingredients:

- 1 large cucumber, sliced
- 10 mint leaves
- Juice of 1 lime
- 4 cups cold water

Preparation:

1. In a large pitcher, combine cucumber slices, mint leaves, and lime juice.
2. Fill with cold water and stir gently.
3. Let it sit in the refrigerator for at least 1 hour to infuse flavors.
4. Serve chilled with ice if desired.

How to Use: Stay hydrated by drinking throughout the day, especially in warm weather and after physical activity.

Coconut Water with Lime Juice Hydration

Intended Use: restores electrolytes and bodily fluids that are naturally lost during exercise or regular activities.

Ingredients:

- Two cups coconut water
- One lime juice
- One tbsp honey or maple syrup (optional)
- One-half tsp sea salt

Preparation:

1. Put sea salt, fresh lime juice, and coconut water in a big pitcher.
2. If you like it sweeter, stir in honey or maple syrup.
3. Thoroughly stir until every component dissolves.
4. Serve right away over ice or refrigerate until cooled.

How to Use: In order to keep hydrated and preserve electrolyte balance, drink one or two glasses after working out or at any point during the day.

Electrolyte Tea with Ginger and Honey

Intended Use: calms the stomach and gives you a rapid energy boost and plenty of water.

Ingredients:

- 1 inch fresh ginger root, thinly sliced
- 4 cups water
- Juice of ½ lemon
- 1 tbsp honey
- A pinch of sea salt

Preparation:

1. Boil water and add ginger slices. Simmer for 10 minutes.
2. Remove from heat and add lemon juice, honey, and a pinch of sea salt. Stir until dissolved.
3. Strain into a pitcher or container and let it cool.

How to Use: Consume warm or chilled, especially during or after illness, to rehydrate and replenish the body.

Drink with Alkalizing Lemon and Apple Cider Vinegar

Intended Use: has an alkalizing impact that improves hydration and pH balance in the body.

Ingredients:

- 2 tbsp apple cider vinegar
- Juice of 1 lemon
- 1 tbsp honey
- 4 cups water

Preparation:

1. In a pitcher, combine apple cider vinegar, lemon juice, and honey.
2. Add water and stir until well mixed and honey is dissolved.
3. Chill in the refrigerator or serve over ice.

How to Use: Have a glass first thing in the morning to aid with digestion and encourage the body to be in an alkaline state.

Golden Milk for Sleep and Hydration

Intended Use: soothes and hydrates the body in preparation for sleep, promoting regeneration during the night.

Ingredients:

- 1 cup almond milk
- ½ tsp turmeric powder
- ¼ tsp cinnamon
- ¼ tsp ginger powder
- A pinch of black pepper
- Honey to taste

Preparation:

1. Heat almond milk in a saucepan over low heat.
2. Whisk in turmeric, cinnamon, ginger, and black pepper.
3. Remove from heat just before boiling.
4. Stir in honey to taste.

5. Serve warm.

How to Use: Thirty minutes before going to bed, have a cup of golden milk to help with hydration and encourage peaceful sleep.

INFLAMMATION REDUCTION

Avocado Salsa with Salmon

Intended Use: Avocados provide good fats, and salmon is rich in omega-3 fatty acids.

Ingredients:

- Two fillets of salmon
- One diced ripe avocado
- One little red onion, cut finely
- one lime's juice
- two tablespoons of finely chopped cilantro
- Pepper, salt, and olive oil

Preparation:

1. Salmon fillets can be baked or grilled with a little salt, pepper, and olive oil.
2. To make the salsa, combine the avocado, red onion, cilantro, and lime juice.
3. Top the salmon with avocado salsa and serve.

Berry and Spinach Smoothie

Intended Use: Antioxidants, which are abundant in berries and spinach, help to reduce inflammation.

Ingredients:

- one cup of raw spinach
- ½ cup of mixed berries, including raspberries, blueberries, and strawberries
- One banana
- One cup almond milk
- One-third tsp flaxseed meal

Preparation:

1. Mix every item until it's smooth.
2. Serve right away.

Black bean and Quinoa Salad

Intended Use: Quinoa and black beans are excellent providers of fiber and plant-based protein.

Ingredients:

- 1 cup cooked black beans, 1 cup cooked quinoa
- One sliced red bell pepper
- 1/4 cup of finely chopped red onion
- 1/4 cup of finely chopped cilantro
- one lime's juice
- Pepper, salt, and olive oil

Preparation:

1. Add the black beans, cilantro, bell pepper, and onion to the quinoa.
2. Add salt, pepper, olive oil, and lime juice to the dressing.

Baked Pears with Ginger

Intended Use: Ginger has anti-inflammatory qualities, while pears are a healthy source of fiber.

Ingredients:

- 4 cored and halved pears
- two tsp finely chopped ginger
- two tsp honey
- half a cup of chopped walnuts
- Arrange the pear halves on a baking sheet

Preparation:

1. Add some ginger and pour some honey on top.
2. Bake for 20 to 25 minutes at 350°F/175°C.
3. Before serving, sprinkle chopped walnuts on top.

Almond and Broccoli Soup

Intended Use: Known for its anti-inflammatory qualities, broccoli is a cruciferous vegetable.

Ingredients:

- Two cups of florets of broccoli

- One sliced onion and two minced garlic cloves
- Four cups of broth made with vegetables
- Half a cup of roasted almonds
- Pepper, salt, and olive oil

Preparation:

1. Garlic and onion are sautéed in olive oil. Sauté the broccoli for a short while.
2. Boil the broth after adding it. Simmer broccoli until it becomes soft.
3. Smoothly blend soup with almonds. Add pepper and salt for seasoning.

Hash with Sweet Potato and Kale

Intended Use: Foods high in nutrients that reduce inflammation include kale and sweet potatoes.

Ingredients:

- 2 medium-sized chopped sweet potatoes
- two cups of finely chopped kale
- One chopped onion
- two minced garlic cloves
- Pepper, salt, and olive oil

Preparation:

1. Garlic and onion should be sautéed in olive oil until transparent.
2. Cook the sweet potatoes until they become soft.
3. Add kale and stir until wilted. Add pepper and salt for seasoning.

Tea with Ginger and Turmeric

Intended Use: Well-known for their anti-inflammatory and antioxidant qualities are ginger and turmeric.

Ingredients:

- 1 inch of freshly grated turmeric root
- One inch of freshly grated ginger root
- One tablespoon of honey
- Juice from one-half lemon

- two cups of water

Preparation:

1. Boil water for ten to fifteen minutes with ginger and turmeric.
2. In a cup, strain the tea.
3. Incorporate the lemon juice and honey. Mix well and serve hot.

Orange and Beet Salad

Intended Use: Rich in vitamins and antioxidants are beets and oranges.

Ingredients:

- 3 medium-sized sliced and roasted beets
- Two peeled and segmented oranges
- 1/4 cup of feta cheese, crumbled
- 1/4 cup of walnuts, chopped
- Balsamic vinegar and olive oil for dressing

Preparation:

1. Place orange segments and beet slices on a platter.
2. Add walnuts and feta cheese on top.
3. Drizzle with balsamic vinegar and olive oil.

Pasta with Walnut and Arugula Pesto

Intended Use: Arugula is a powerhouse of antioxidants, while walnuts are a fantastic source of omega-3s.

Ingredients:

- half a cup of walnuts
- Two cups of arugula
- Grated Parmesan cheese, half a cup
- half a cup of olive oil
- two garlic cloves
- To taste, add salt and pepper.
- pasta made with whole grains

Preparation:

1. In a food processor, pulse walnuts, arugula, Parmesan, garlic, and olive oil until smooth.
2. Follow the directions on the package to cook the pasta. After draining, combine with pesto.

Pineapple and Cherry Anti-Inflammatory Drink

Intended Use: combines the anti-inflammatory properties of bromelain- and anthocyanin-rich pineapple with the benefits of cherries.

Ingredients:

- 1 cup tart cherry juice
- 1 cup pineapple chunks
- 1 tsp honey (optional)
- Water or ice as needed

Preparation:

1. Blend cherry juice and pineapple chunks until smooth.
2. Add honey for sweetness if desired.
3. Adjust consistency with water or ice.
4. Serve chilled.

How to Use: Drink once a day to help decrease inflammation and discomfort in the muscles, especially after working out.

Mixed Berries with Chia Seed Pudding

Intended Use: Antioxidants abound in berries, and chia seeds are strong in omega-3 fatty acids.

Ingredients:

- 1/4 cup of chia seeds.
- One cup coconut milk
- One tablespoon of honey
- Half a cup of mixed berries

Preparation:

1. In a bowl, combine honey, coconut milk, and chia seeds. Allow to rest for the

night.
2. Before serving, sprinkle mixed berries on top.

Mint with Cucumber Water

Intended Use: Cucumber lends a refreshing twist to water, which is beneficial for reducing inflammation.

Ingredients:

- One cucumber, cut thinly
- ten mint leaves
- One water liter

Preparation:

1. Put all the ingredients into a big pitcher.
2. To bring out the flavors, refrigerate for at least an hour before serving.

Roasted Cauliflower with Turmeric

Intended Use: The anti-inflammatory properties of both turmeric and cauliflower are well-known.

Ingredients:

- One head of chopped cauliflower
- Two tsp olive oil
- One tsp of turmeric
- To taste, add salt and pepper.

Preparation:

1. Combine olive oil, turmeric, salt, and pepper with the cauliflower florets.
2. Roast for 25 to 30 minutes at 400°F (200°C) or until soft and brown.

Tomato Salad and Avocado

Intended Use: Tomatoes are abundant in antioxidants while avocados are rich in monounsaturated fats.

Ingredients:

- 1/4 cup finely chopped red onion,
- 2 diced tomatoes, and
- 2 ripe avocados
- one lime's juice
- To taste, add salt and pepper.

Preparation:

1. Mix the avocados, tomatoes, and red onion together in a bowl.
2. Add pepper, salt, and lime juice for dressing.

Quinoa with spinach and mushrooms

Intended Use: Rich in vitamins, quinoa offers a complete protein, while mushrooms have anti-inflammatory properties.

Ingredients:

- 1 cup cooked quinoa,
- 2 cups wilted spinach,
- 1 cup sautéed mushrooms, and
- 1 minced garlic clove.
- Pepper, salt, and olive oil

Preparation:

1. Add olive oil and sauté the garlic and mushrooms. Cook the spinach until it begins to wilt.
2. Mix the cooked quinoa with the vegetables. Add pepper and salt for seasoning.

Herb-and-Lemon Baked Cod

Intended Use: Lemon offers vitamin C, while fish like cod are lean protein sources.

Ingredients:

- Four fillets of cod
- One lemon's juice
- One tablespoon of olive oil
- One tspn dry herbs (basil, oregano, and thyme)
- To taste, add salt and pepper.

Preparation:

1. Cod should be marinated with lemon juice, olive oil, herbs, and seasonings.
2. Fish should flake readily after 12 to 15 minutes of baking at 375°F (190°C).

Ginger-Turmeric Anti-Inflammatory Tea

Intended Use: uses ginger's and turmeric's anti-inflammatory qualities to reduce pain and inflammation.

Ingredients:

- 1 tsp turmeric powder
- 1 tsp grated fresh ginger
- 1 tsp black pepper (to enhance turmeric absorption)
- 1 tbsp honey (optional)
- 2 cups water

Preparation:

1. Boil water in a pot. Add turmeric and ginger.
2. Simmer for 10 minutes. Add black pepper.
3. Strain the mixture into a cup.
4. Add honey to taste and stir well.

How to Use: Drink one or two glasses every day, particularly if you're feeling irritated or uncomfortable.

Rich Flaxseed Smoothie with Omega-3

Intended Use: high quantities of Omega-3 fatty acids from flaxseeds support the lowering of overall inflammation.

Ingredients:

- 2 tbsp ground flaxseed
- 1 banana
- 1 cup spinach
- ½ cup blueberries
- 1 cup almond milk

Preparation:

1. Place all ingredients in a blender.
2. Blend until smooth.
3. Serve immediately.

How to Use: Start your day with this smoothie for breakfast or as a snack to get more anti-inflammatory elements in your diet.

Aloe Vera and Anti-Inflammatory Cucumber Gel

Intended Use: topically lowers skin irritation and inflammation because to the cooling properties of cucumber and aloe vera.

Ingredients:

- ¼ cup aloe vera gel
- ¼ cup cucumber juice
- 1 tbsp coconut oil
- A few drops of lavender essential oil

Preparation:

1. Blend fresh cucumber to make juice, then strain.
2. Mix aloe vera gel, cucumber juice, and coconut oil.
3. Add lavender essential oil and stir well.
4. Store in a glass jar in the refrigerator.

How to Use: To reduce inflammation, apply to afflicted skin regions two to three times a day, or as needed.

Anti-Inflammatory Paste with Rosemary and Basil

Intended Use: The anti-inflammatory qualities of rosemary and basil reduce pain and inflammation.

Ingredients:

- ½ cup fresh basil leaves
- ¼ cup fresh rosemary leaves
- 2-3 tbsp olive oil

Preparation:

1. Blend basil and rosemary leaves with olive oil to create a paste.

2. If needed, adjust the consistency by adding more olive oil.
3. Store in an airtight container in the refrigerator.

How to Use: Once or twice a day, gently massage painful or inflammatory regions.

Leafy green vegetable salad with a dressing that reduces inflammation

Intended Use: reduces inflammation by eating a diet high in green leafy vegetables, which are high in antioxidants.

Ingredients for Salad:

- 2 cups mixed greens (spinach, kale, arugula)
- ½ avocado, sliced
- ¼ cup walnuts

Ingredients for Dressing:

- 2 tbsp extra virgin olive oil
- 1 tbsp apple cider vinegar
- 1 tsp Dijon mustard
- 1 tsp honey
- Salt and pepper to taste

Preparation:

1. Combine salad ingredients in a large bowl.
2. Whisk together dressing ingredients in a small bowl.
3. Pour dressing over salad and toss gently.

How to Use: Enjoy this salad regularly, ideally as part of your daily meals, to benefit from its anti-inflammatory effects.

Juice from Celery for Inflammation

Intended Use: Celery's inherent anti-inflammatory properties help to reduce inflammation and aid in the body's detoxification.

Ingredients:

- 1 bunch of celery, washed and chopped

Preparation:

1. Run celery through a juicer to extract juice.
2. Drink fresh celery juice immediately for best nutritional benefits.

How to Use: For maximum anti-inflammatory benefits, take 16 ounces of celery juice first thing in the morning on an empty stomach.

Sprouting Fenugreek Seeds

Intended Use: Reduces external inflammation and soothes pain with the anti-inflammatory properties of fenugreek seeds.

Ingredients:

- ¼ cup fenugreek seeds
- Warm water

Preparation:

1. Grind fenugreek seeds into a fine powder.
2. Mix fenugreek powder with enough warm water to form a thick paste.
3. Apply directly to the inflamed area.
4. Cover with a cloth and let sit for 1-2 hours.
5. Rinse off with warm water.

How to Use: Apply once a day to afflicted areas to lessen pain and inflammation.

Black pepper with turmeric pills

Intended Use: improves curcumin absorption when combined with black pepper and has systemic anti-inflammatory properties.

Ingredients:

- Turmeric powder
- Ground black pepper
- Empty capsules

Preparation:

1. Mix turmeric powder with a small amount of ground black pepper (a 10:1 ratio of turmeric to pepper is recommended).
2. Fill empty capsules with the mixture using a small spoon or a capsule filling

machine.
3. Store in a cool, dry place.

How to Use: Take one or two capsules with meals every day to help support the body's overall decrease of inflammation.

Bone Broth with Anti-Inflammation

Intended Use: improves intestinal health and lowers inflammation because to bone broth's restorative qualities—it's high in collagen and minerals.

Ingredients:

- 2 pounds mixed bones (chicken, beef, fish)
- 2 carrots, chopped
- 1 onion, chopped
- 2 stalks celery, chopped
- 2 tbsp apple cider vinegar
- Water to cover
- Herbs and spices (optional: garlic, bay leaves, thyme)

Preparation:

1. Place bones in a large pot and cover with water. Add apple cider vinegar.
2. Bring to a boil, then reduce heat and simmer for 12-24 hours. Skim off any foam that forms on the surface.
3. Add vegetables and optional herbs in the last few hours of cooking.
4. Strain the broth through a fine mesh sieve, discarding solids.
5. Store broth in the refrigerator or freezer.

How to Use: Every day, drink one cup of warm bone broth, particularly when you're experiencing more physical stress or inflammation.

COMBINED ADAPTABILITY AND MOBILITY

Rich Flaxseed Smoothie with Omega-3

Intended Use: utilizes the Omega-3 fatty acids found in flaxseeds to improve joint flexibility and lower inflammation.

Ingredients:

- 2 tbsp ground flaxseed
- 1 banana
- 1 cup spinach
- ½ cup blueberries
- 1 cup almond milk

Preparation:

1. Place all ingredients in a blender.
2. Blend until smooth.
3. Serve immediately for the best nutrient retention.

How to Use: Drink this smoothie every day to add Omega-3 fats, which reduce inflammation, to your diet.

A Walnut and Avocado Salad for Healthy Joints

Intended Use: Supports joint health with healthy fats from avocados and walnuts, known for their anti-inflammatory properties.

Ingredients:

- 2 cups mixed greens
- 1 ripe avocado, sliced
- ½ cup walnuts, roughly chopped
- Dressing: 2 tbsp olive oil, 1 tbsp apple cider vinegar, salt, and pepper

Preparation:

1. In a large salad bowl, combine mixed greens, avocado slices, and walnuts.
2. In a small bowl, whisk together olive oil, apple cider vinegar, salt, and pepper to create the dressing.

3. Drizzle the dressing over the salad and toss gently to combine.

How to Use: To reap the benefits of its joint-supporting ingredients, eat this salad often.

Cherry Juice for Improved Joint Flexibility

Intended Use: uses the anthocyanins present in cherries to reduce inflammation in the joints and support mobility.

Ingredients:

- 2 cups fresh or frozen cherries
- Water as needed

Preparation:

1. Blend cherries with a little water until smooth.
2. Strain the mixture to remove solid particles and extract juice.
3. Serve the juice chilled or at room temperature.

How to Use: Have a glass of cherry juice every day to help increase flexibility and lessen pain in your joints, especially after working out.

Infusion of Stinging Nettle for Joint Health

Intended Use: Rich in minerals and vitamins, stinging nettle supports joint health by reducing inflammation.

Ingredients:

- 1 cup dried stinging nettle leaves
- 4 cups boiling water

Preparation:

1. Place nettle leaves in a large jar.
2. Pour boiling water over the leaves.
3. Cover and steep for 4 hours or overnight.
4. Strain and store the infusion in the refrigerator.

How to Use: Every day, consume one to two cups of nettle infusion to promote joint health and flexibility.

Ginger-Turmeric Joint Health Tea

Intended Use: Due to the anti-inflammatory qualities of ginger and turmeric, it reduces joint discomfort and increases flexibility.

Ingredients:

- 1 tsp turmeric powder
- 1 tsp grated fresh ginger
- 1 tsp black pepper (to enhance absorption of turmeric)
- 1 tbsp honey (optional)
- 2 cups water

Preparation:

1. Boil water in a pot. Add turmeric and ginger.
2. Simmer for 10 minutes. Add black pepper.
3. Strain the mixture into a cup.
4. Add honey to taste and stir well.

How to Use: Have one to two cups per day to help with inflammation reduction and joint health.

Bone Broth for Flexible Joints

Intended Use: Supports joint health and flexibility with the collagen and minerals found in bone broth.

Ingredients:

- 2 pounds mixed bones (beef, chicken, or fish)
- 2 carrots, chopped
- 1 onion, chopped
- 2 stalks celery, chopped
- 2 tbsp apple cider vinegar
- Water to cover
- Herbs and spices (optional)

Preparation:

1. Place bones in a large pot and cover with water. Add apple cider vinegar.
2. Bring to a boil, then reduce heat and simmer for 12-24 hours. Skim off any foam that

forms on the surface.
3. Add vegetables and optional herbs in the last few hours of cooking.
4. Strain the broth through a fine mesh sieve, discarding solids.
5. Store broth in the refrigerator or freezer.

How to Use: Every day, drink one cup of warm bone broth to help lubricate joints and increase flexibility.

Stretching with Herbal Muscle Rub and Yoga

Intended Use: A DIY herbal massage helps to improve flexibility and relieve tense muscles.

Ingredients:

- ¼ cup coconut oil
- ¼ cup shea butter
- 2 tbsp beeswax
- 10 drops lavender essential oil
- 10 drops peppermint essential oil
- 5 drops eucalyptus essential oil

Preparation:

1. Melt coconut oil, shea butter, and beeswax in a double boiler.
2. Remove from heat and let cool slightly.
3. Stir in essential oils.
4. Pour into a container and let solidify.

How to Use: Apply to tight joints and muscles to increase flexibility and reduce pain, both before and after yoga or stretching activities.

Smoothie with Pineapple and Turmeric Anti-Inflammatory

Intended Use: uses turmeric and bromelain from pineapple to help reduce inflammation and increase joint mobility.

Ingredients:

- 1 cup pineapple chunks
- 1 tsp turmeric powder
- ½ tsp black pepper

- 1 cup coconut water
- 1 tbsp chia seeds

Preparation:

1. Place pineapple, turmeric, black pepper, coconut water, and chia seeds in a blender.
2. Blend until smooth.
3. Serve immediately.

How to Use: Regular consumption of this smoothie, particularly after exercise, will help to maintain joint health and lower inflammation.

Omega-3 salad with salmon and walnuts

Intended Use: uses Omega-3 fatty acids from walnuts and salmon to improve joint flexibility and lower inflammation.

Ingredients:

- 2 cups mixed greens
- 4 ounces cooked salmon, flaked
- ¼ cup walnuts, chopped
- Dressing: 2 tbsp olive oil,
- 1 tbsp lemon juice, salt, and pepper

Preparation:

1. Arrange mixed greens on a plate.
2. Top with flaked salmon and chopped walnuts.
3. In a small bowl, whisk together olive oil, lemon juice, salt, and pepper.
4. Drizzle dressing over the salad.

How to Use: Incorporate this salad into your meals 2-3 times a week to benefit from the anti-inflammatory and joint-supporting properties of Omega- 3 fatty acids.

RELIEF FOR JOINTS AND MUSCLE

Turmeric and Ginger Anti-Inflammatory Tea

Intended Use: Reduces inflammation and soothes muscle pain with the potent anti-inflammatory properties of ginger and turmeric.

Ingredients:

- 1 inch fresh ginger root, thinly sliced
- 1 tsp turmeric powder or 1 inch turmeric root, thinly sliced
- Juice of ½ lemon
- 1 tbsp honey (optional)
- 4 cups boiling water

Preparation:

1. Place ginger and turmeric in a pot and cover with boiling water.
2. Let simmer for 10-15 minutes.
3. Strain the tea into mugs, adding lemon juice and honey to each for flavor.
4. Stir well before drinking.

How to Use: To assist with joint and muscle relaxation, especially after physical exertion, consume one to two cups per day.

Epsom Salt and Lavender Oil Bath Soak

Intended Use: Epsom salt's muscle-relaxing qualities combined with the calming aroma of lavender help to relax muscles and lessen stiffness and soreness.

Ingredients:

- 2 cups Epsom salt
- 10 drops lavender essential oil
- Warm bathwater

Preparation:

1. Fill your bathtub with warm water.
2. Dissolve Epsom salt in the bathwater.
3. Add lavender essential oil and swirl the water to mix.

4. Soak in the bath for 20-30 minutes.

How to Use: Take this soothing bath soak two or three times a week, especially after days when you've been physically strained or when you have aching muscles.

Muscle rub with coconut oil and cayenne pepper

Intended Use: increases circulation by using the capsaicin in cayenne pepper to provide warming relief for tense muscles and joint discomfort.

Ingredients:

- ¼ cup coconut oil
- 1 tbsp cayenne pepper powder
- Glass jar for storage

Preparation:

1. Gently melt coconut oil in a double boiler.
2. Remove from heat and mix in the cayenne pepper powder thoroughly.
3. Pour the mixture into a glass jar and allow it to cool and solidify.
4. Apply a small amount to sore areas, being careful to avoid sensitive skin and eyes.

How to Use: Apply gently, no more than twice a day, to afflicted areas. First, do a patch test on a tiny section of skin to make sure there is no irritation.

Tea Made with Natural Willow Bark Pain Relieving

Intended Use: Willow bark, which has a high salicin concentration, provides a natural pain relief solution for aches and pains in the muscles and joints.

Ingredients:

- 1 tsp dried willow bark
- 2 cups water

Preparation:

1. Boil water in a pot and add willow bark.
2. Reduce heat and simmer for 10-15 minutes.
3. Strain the tea into a cup and let it cool slightly before drinking.

How to Use: Sip one cup of willow bark tea up to twice a day if you have discomfort in your muscles or joints. If you are on blood thinners or are allergic to aspirin, speak with your doctor before using.

Arnica and Lavender Soothing Balm for Muscles

Intended Use: uses the relaxing qualities of lavender and the anti-inflammatory qualities of arnica to relieve joint pain and tired muscles.

Ingredients:

- ½ cup coconut oil
- 2 tbsp beeswax pellets
- ¼ cup arnica oil
- 20 drops lavender essential oil
- Small jar or tin for storage

Preparation:

1. Melt coconut oil and beeswax together in a double boiler over low heat.
2. Once melted, remove from heat and stir in the arnica oil.
3. Allow the mixture to cool slightly before adding the lavender essential oil, stirring well to combine.
4. Pour into your chosen container and let it set until solid.

How to Use: As needed, apply a tiny quantity of the balm on achy joints or muscles. Steer clear of sensitive or damaged skin regions.

Eucalyptus and Peppermint Muscle Soothing Spray

Intended Use: provides immediate relief from tense and painful muscles thanks to the calming properties of eucalyptus and peppermint.

Ingredients:

- ¼ cup witch hazel
- 10 drops peppermint essential oil
- 10 drops eucalyptus essential oil
- ½ cup distilled water
- Spray bottle

Preparation:

1. In a spray bottle, combine witch hazel, distilled water, peppermint,

2. and eucalyptus essential oils.
3. Shake well to mix.
4. Spray directly onto sore muscles as needed, avoiding the face and sensitive areas.

How to Use: For cooling relief, apply to afflicted muscles two to three times a day or after activity.

Beetroot and Cherry Juice for Restoring Muscle

Intended Use: Antioxidants from beets and cherries aid in muscle repair and minimize inflammation after exercise.

Ingredients:

- 1 cup fresh or frozen cherries
- 1 medium beetroot, peeled and diced
- Water or coconut water, as needed for blending

Preparation:

1. Blend cherries and beetroot together, adding just enough water or coconut water to achieve a smooth consistency.
2. Strain the mixture if desired for a smoother juice.
3. Drink immediately or store in the refrigerator for up to 24 hours.

How to Use: Take within half an hour after working out to help reduce inflammation and help muscles recover.

Healing Bath Salts with Mint and Rosemary

Intended Use: Soothes muscle aches and improves circulation with the therapeutic properties of rosemary and mint.

Ingredients:

- 1 cup Epsom salt
- ½ cup sea salt
- 10 drops rosemary essential oil
- 10 drops peppermint essential oil
- Dried rosemary and mint leaves (optional)

Preparation:

1. In a bowl, mix Epsom salt and sea salt together.
2. Add essential oils and dried herbs, if using, and mix well.
3. Store in an airtight container.
4. Add ½ to 1 cup of the salt mixture to warm bathwater.

How to Use: To ease the pain in your muscles and joints, soak in the bathtub for at least 20 minutes.

Smoothie with Moringa Leaf Powder to Build Muscle

Intended Use: Enhances muscle strength and flexibility with the high nutritional content of moringa leaf powder.

Ingredients:

- 1 tsp moringa leaf powder
- 1 banana
- ½ cup spinach
- 1 cup almond milk
- 1 tbsp almond butter

Preparation:

1. Place all ingredients in a blender.
2. Blend until smooth.
3. Serve immediately for the best flavor and nutrient benefits.

How to Use: Consume this smoothie to enhance muscular health and vitality in the morning or after working out.

Infusion of Stinging Nettle for Joint Pain Relief

Intended Use: Alleviates joint pain and supports muscle health with the nutrient-rich properties of stinging nettle.

Ingredients:

- 1 cup dried stinging nettle leaves
- 4 cups boiling water

Preparation:

1. Place stinging nettle leaves in a large jar or pot.

2. Pour boiling water over the leaves and cover.
3. Let steep for 4 hours or overnight for a strong infusion.
4. Strain and store the liquid in the refrigerator.

How to Use: Take one cup of nettle infusion each day, or blend it into smoothies.

KIDNEY ASSISTANT

Lemon Water with Parsley

Intended Use: improves renal function and eliminates toxins from the body through the purifying properties of lemon and parsley.

Ingredients:

- A handful of fresh parsley
- Juice of 1 lemon
- 1 liter of water

Preparation:

1. Rinse the parsley and chop it roughly.
2. Add chopped parsley and lemon juice to a liter of water.
3. Let it infuse overnight in the refrigerator.
4. Strain and drink the water throughout the next day.

How to Use: Consume daily to aid kidney function and improve urinary tract health.

Kidney Cleanse Juice with Cranberries

Intended Use: Prevents urinary tract infections and supports kidney health with the antibacterial properties of cranberries.

Ingredients:

- 1 cup fresh or unsweetened cranberries
- 2 cups water
- 1 tbsp honey (optional)

Preparation:

1. Blend cranberries with water until smooth.
2. Strain the mixture to remove solid particles.
3. Sweeten with honey if desired.
4. Serve chilled.

How to Use: Have a glass of cranberry juice every day to help kidney cleaning and urinary tract health.

Root Tea with Dandelion

Intended Use: provides natural diuretic benefits to support kidney function and cleansing.

Ingredients:

- 1 tbsp dried dandelion root
- 1 cup boiling water

Preparation:

1. Place dandelion root in a tea infuser or directly in a mug.
2. Pour boiling water over the dandelion root and cover.
3. Steep for 10 minutes.
4. Strain and enjoy the tea warm.

How to Use: To assist kidney health and encourage natural detoxification, consume one to two cups each day.

Infusion of Nettle Leaf

Intended Use: nourishes and diuretes the body with nettle leaves, supporting kidney health and boosting urine output.

Ingredients:

- 1 cup dried nettle leaves
- 1 liter boiling water

Preparation:

1. Place nettle leaves in a large jar.
2. Pour boiling water over the leaves.
3. Cover and let steep for 4-6 hours or overnight.
4. Strain the infusion and store in the refrigerator.

How to Use: For optimal kidney function and cleansing, consume one to two cups of nettle leaf infusion on a daily basis.

Hydration Drink with Watermelon

Intended Use: Watermelon's natural diuretic characteristics hydrate and cleanse the kidneys.

Ingredients:

- 2 cups cubed watermelon
- 1 cup coconut water
- Juice of 1 lime

Preparation:

1. Blend watermelon, coconut water, and lime juice until smooth.
2. Serve immediately, optionally over ice.

How to Use: Enjoy this cool beverage to help maintain kidney health and hydration on hot days or after working out.

Herbal Supplements for Kidney Support

Intended Use: combines a variety of kidney-supporting herbs to promote kidney function and health.

Ingredients:

- Dried herbs: burdock root, uva ursi, and juniper berries (in equal parts)
- Empty capsules

Preparation:

1. Finely grind the dried herbs together to a powder.
2. Fill empty capsules with the herbal mixture using a capsule machine or a small spoon.
3. Store the capsules in a cool, dry place.

How to Use: Take 1-2 capsules daily with plenty of water to support kidney health. Consult a healthcare provider before use, especially if you have kidney disease or are pregnant.

Smoothie for Kidney Cleanse with Celery and Apple

Intended Use: helps remove kidney toxins and has anti-inflammatory properties when combined with apple and celery.

Ingredients:

- 2 stalks of celery
- 1 green apple, cored and sliced
- ½ cup parsley leaves
- 1 cup water or coconut water
- Juice of ½ lemon

Preparation:

1. Combine all ingredients in a blender.
2. Blend until smooth.
3. Serve immediately for maximum freshness and nutrient content.

How to Use: with the morning, have this smoothie on an empty stomach to aid with kidney cleaning and general well-being.

Kidney detox salad with cucumber and beets

Intended Use: utilizes nutrient-dense beets and cucumber to support kidney health and cleansing.

Ingredients:

- 1 medium beet, grated
- 1 cucumber, thinly sliced
- Dressing: olive oil, lemon juice, salt, and pepper to taste
- Fresh herbs (optional): parsley or dill

Preparation:

1. Combine grated beet and sliced cucumber in a salad bowl.
2. Prepare the dressing by whisking together olive oil, lemon juice, salt,and pepper.
3. Drizzle the dressing over the salad and toss gently.
4. Garnish with fresh herbs if desired.

How to Use: Incorporate this salad into your meals 2-3 times a week forkidney support and detoxification.

Tea with Goldenrod Flavor

Intended Use: Relieves inflammation of the urinary tract and supports kidney health with the anti-inflammatory properties of goldenrod.

Ingredients:

- 1 tsp dried goldenrod flowers
- 1 cup boiling water

Preparation:

1. Place goldenrod flowers in a tea infuser or directly in a cup.
2. Pour boiling water over the flowers.
3. Cover and steep for about 10 minutes.
4. Strain and drink the tea warm.

How to Use: To promote kidney function and urinary tract health, have one cup of goldenrod tea every day.

Barley Water for Healthy Kidneys

Intended Use: barley's diuretic qualities help to clear out toxins and support kidney function.

Ingredients:

- ¼ cup pearl barley
- 4 cups water
- Lemon juice and honey to taste

Preparation:

1. Rinse barley under cold water.
2. Combine barley and water in a pot and bring to a boil.
3. Reduce heat and simmer for 30 minutes.
4. Strain and add lemon juice and honey to taste.
5. Serve warm or chilled.

How to Use: To maintain urinary tract function and kidney health, have a cup of barley water every day.

HEALTH OF LIVER

Beet Juice for Liver Cleansing

Intended Use: helps the body detoxify the liver and boosts antioxidant levels with beetroot.

Ingredients:

- 2 medium beets, peeled and chopped
- 1 green apple, chopped
- 1-inch piece of fresh ginger, peeled
- ½ lemon, peeled
- 1 cup water

Preparation:

1. Combine all ingredients in a blender.
2. Blend until smooth.
3. Strain the mixture to extract the juice.
4. Serve the juice immediately or chill for an hour before drinking.

How to Use: For the purpose of supporting liver health and promoting detoxification, have one glass of beet juice every morning.

Drink with Lemon Liver Flush and Turmeric

Intended Use: Stimulates liver function and provides anti-inflammatory benefits with turmeric and lemon.

Ingredients:

- 1 tsp turmeric powder
- Juice of 1 lemon
- 1 cup warm water
- 1 tsp honey (optional)

Preparation:

1. Dissolve turmeric powder and lemon juice in warm water.
2. Add honey for sweetness, if desired.
3. Stir well until all ingredients are well combined.

How to Use: Drink on an empty stomach each morning to stimulate liver detoxification and reduce inflammation.

Milk Thistle Tea

Intended Use: Because of its silymarin concentration, milk thistle supports liver function and protects liver cells.

Ingredients:

- 1 tbsp milk thistle seeds
- 2 cups boiling water

Preparation:

1. Crush milk thistle seeds slightly to release silymarin.
2. Place seeds in a teapot or heat-proof container.
3. Pour boiling water over seeds and steep for 20 minutes.
4. Strain and serve the tea warm.

How to Use: For daily liver protection and function support, have one cup of milk thistle tea.

Tea Made with Dandelion Detox

Intended Use: Supports liver detoxification and health with dandelion root, known for its liver-supportive properties.

Ingredients:

- 2 tbsp dried dandelion root
- 4 cups boiling water
- Lemon slice and honey (optional)

Preparation:

1. Place dandelion root in a pot and cover with boiling water.
2. Simmer for 10-15 minutes.
3. Strain the tea into cups.
4. Add a slice of lemon and honey to taste, if desired.

How to Use: Sip one to two glasses daily, preferably first thing in the morning, to aid in the generation of bile and liver cleansing.

Smoothie for Healthy Liver

Intended Use: combines a variety of greens that are good for the liver to provide vital nutrients for liver health.

Ingredients:

- 1 cup spinach
- 1 cup kale, stems removed
- 1 apple, cored and chopped
- ½ cucumber, chopped
- 1 tbsp chia seeds
- 1 cup water or coconut water

Preparation:

1. Place all ingredients in a blender.
2. Blend on high until smooth.
3. Serve immediately for the best taste and nutrient retention.

How to Use: Enjoy this smoothie daily as a nutritious breakfast or snack to support overall liver health.

Liver tonic with apple cider vinegar

Intended Use: uses apple cider vinegar to enhance digestion and support liver cleansing.

Ingredients:

- 2 tbsp organic apple cider vinegar
- 1 tbsp honey
- 1 cup warm water

Preparation:

1. Dissolve honey in warm water in a glass.
2. Add apple cider vinegar and stir well.
3. Consume the mixture.

How to Use: To promote liver health and facilitate digestion, take one serving of this tonic each day, ideally first thing in the morning on an empty stomach.

Walnut and Avocado Liver Health Salad

Intended Use: Supports liver health with healthy fats from avocado and walnuts, plus detoxifying greens.

Ingredients:

- 2 cups mixed salad greens
- 1 ripe avocado, diced
- ½ cup walnuts, roughly chopped
- Dressing: Juice of 1 lemon,
- 2 tbsp olive oil, salt, and pepper

Preparation:

1. Toss salad greens, diced avocado, and walnuts in a large salad bowl.
2. In a small bowl, whisk together lemon juice, olive oil, salt, and pepper to make the dressing.
3. Drizzle dressing over the salad and toss gently to combine.

How to Use: Include this salad in your diet two or three times a week to provide your liver the nutrition and good fats it needs.

Artichoke Heart Detox Tea for Liver

Intended Use: aids in liver cleansing and bile generation with artichoke hearts, known for their cynarin content.

Ingredients:

- 2 fresh or canned artichoke hearts
- 4 cups water
- Lemon slice (optional)

Preparation:

1. If using fresh artichoke hearts, rinse and chop them.
2. Boil artichoke hearts in water for 15 minutes.
3. Strain the tea and add a slice of lemon if desired.
4. Serve warm or chilled.

How to Use: Every day, consume one cup of artichoke heart tea to promote bile production and liver function.

Liver Support Herbal Capsules

Intended Use: offers a practical method of ingesting a combination of herbs that help the liver.

Ingredients:

- Dried herbs: dandelion root,
- burdock root,
- turmeric root, and
- milkthistle seed (in equal parts)
- Empty capsules

Preparation:

1. Finely powder the dried herbs using a coffee grinder or mortar andpestle.
2. Mix the powdered herbs thoroughly.
3. Use a capsule machine or a small spoon to fill empty capsules withthe herbal mixture.
4. Store the filled capsules in a cool, dry place.

How to Use: Take 1-2 capsules with water twice daily, morning and evening,to support liver health and detoxification.

Olive Oil and Garlic Liver Cleanse

Intended Use: Garlic's sulfur-containing components stimulate liver function and aid in detoxification.

Ingredients:

- 1 clove garlic, minced
- 1 tbsp extra virgin olive oil

Preparation:

1. Combine minced garlic with olive oil in a small bowl.
2. Let the mixture sit for 10 minutes to allow the garlic compounds to infuse into the oil.
3. Consume the mixture directly or spread on a small piece of whole- grain bread.

How to Use: To aid with liver cleansing, take one daily dose of this garlic and olive oil combo, ideally in the evening.

IMPROVEMENT OF MOOD

Walnut and Flaxseed Smoothie Packed with Omega-3

Intended Use: provides the omega-3 fatty acids included in walnuts and flaxseeds to support brain function and mood enhancement.

Ingredients:

¼ cup walnuts

1 tbsp ground flaxseed

1 banana

1 cup spinach leaves

1 cup almond milk

Preparation:

Place all ingredients in a blender.

Blend until smooth.

Serve immediately for the best nutrient retention.

How to Use: Enjoy this smoothie in the morning to start your day with a mood boost.

Aromatherapy using Essential Lavender Oil

Intended Use: uses the calming aroma of lavender to provide a sense of serenity and enhanced mood while reducing tension and anxiety.

Ingredients:

Lavender essential oil

Diffuser or cotton ball

Preparation:

Add a few drops of lavender essential oil to a diffuser filled with water and turn it on.

Alternatively, add a few drops to a cotton ball and place it near your workspace or bedside.

How to Use: Keep the scented cotton ball close by for ongoing mood enhancement, or use the diffuser in your living area for at least thirty minutes each day.

The Adaptogenic Tonic of Ashwagandha

Intended Use: Ashwagandha's adaptogenic qualities improve mood and reduce stress.

Ingredients:

½ tsp Ashwagandha powder

1 cup warm milk (dairy or plant-based)

Honey to taste

Preparation:

Mix Ashwagandha powder into warm milk until well dissolved.

Sweeten with honey to taste.

Drink warm before bedtime.

How to Use: Take once a night to help lower stress and elevate mood.

Vivacious Citrus Mood Enhancing Drink

Intended Use: Boosts mood and energy levels with the uplifting properties of citrus fruits.

Ingredients:

Juice of 1 orange

Juice of ½ lemon

1 tsp grated ginger

1 cup cold water or sparkling water

Ice cubes

Honey (optional)

Preparation:

Combine orange juice, lemon juice, and grated ginger in a glass.

Add cold or sparkling water and stir well.

Add ice cubes and sweeten with honey if desired.

How to Use: During the day, sip as needed to instantly improve your mood and give you more energy.

Mood Refreshing Spray with Peppermint

Intended Use: The energizing aroma of peppermint elevates and refreshes the spirit.

Ingredients:

- ½ cup distilled water
- 2 tbsp witch hazel
- 10-15 drops peppermint essential oil
- Spray bottle

Preparation:

1. Combine water and witch hazel in a spray bottle.
2. Add peppermint essential oil and shake well to mix.
3. Spray lightly around your living or workspace.

How to Use: To revive your senses and raise your spirits, use as required.

B Nut-Rich Nut Snack Blend

Intended Use: enhances energy and emotional control with a blend of high-B vitamin nuts.

Ingredients:

- ¼ cup almonds
- ¼ cup walnuts
- ¼ cup sunflower seeds
- ¼ cup pumpkin seeds
- Sea salt (optional)

Preparation:

1. Mix almonds, walnuts, sunflower seeds, and pumpkin seeds in a bowl.
2. Lightly toast the mix in a dry skillet over medium heat until fragrant.
3. Sprinkle with a pinch of sea salt if desired.
4. Let cool before serving.

How to Use: Throughout the day, munch on this mixture to sustain your energy and uplift your spirits.

Tea with Chamomile and St. John's Wort

Intended Use: Reduces mild to moderate anxiety and sadness while enhancing mood overall thanks to St. John's Wort's mood-stabilizing characteristics and chamomile's relaxing effects.

Ingredients:

1 tsp dried St. John's Wort

1 tsp dried chamomile flowers

1 cup boiling water

Honey (optional)

Preparation:

Mix St. John's Wort and chamomile flowers in a tea infuser or directly in a cup.

Pour boiling water over the herbs and cover the cup.

Steep for 5-10 minutes.

Strain the tea into another cup if needed and sweeten with honey if desired.

How to Use: To improve mood and lessen anxiety, drink this tea once a day, especially in the afternoon or evening. Note: There may be drug interactions with St. John's Wort. Before using, speak with a healthcare professional.

Maca Powder Energy Balls

Intended Use: Increases energy and enhances mood with the natural energizing properties of Maca powder.

Ingredients:

1 cup dates, pitted

½ cup almonds

2 tbsp Maca powder

1 tbsp cocoa powder

Shredded coconut for coating

Preparation:

Blend dates and almonds in a food processor until they form a sticky dough.

Add Maca powder and cocoa powder; pulse until well combined.

Roll the mixture into small balls.

Coat each ball in shredded coconut.

Refrigerate for at least an hour before serving.

How to Use: For a mood and energy boost, eat one or two energy balls as needed during the day.

Milk with Saffron and Turmeric

Intended Use: Promotes a positive mood and relaxation with the mood- enhancing properties of saffron and the anti-inflammatory benefits of turmeric.

Ingredients:

1 cup milk (dairy or plant-based)

¼ tsp turmeric powder

A pinch of saffron strands

Honey to taste

Preparation:

Heat milk in a saucepan over low heat.

Add turmeric and saffron; stir until well combined.

Remove from heat and sweeten with honey.

Serve warm.

How to Use: Drink in the evening to unwind and lift your spirits before going to sleep.

Ginseng Tea for Emotional Balance

Intended Use: Improves mental clarity and enhances mood with theadaptogenic effects of ginseng.

Ingredients:

- 1 tsp ginseng root (sliced or powdered)

- 1 cup boiling water

Preparation:

1. Place ginseng in a cup or tea infuser.
2. Pour boiling water over ginseng and cover.
3. Steep for 5-10 minutes.
4. Strain and drink warm.

How to Use: Sip one cup of ginseng tea in the morning to promote mood and mental clarity all day.

HEART SUPPORT

Beet Juice for Liver Cleansing

Intended Use: Enhances liver function and blood purification with the detoxifying benefits of beets.

Ingredients:

- 2 medium beets, peeled and chopped
- 3 carrots, peeled and chopped
- 1 apple, cored and sliced
- ½ lemon, peeled
- 1-inch piece of ginger, peeled

Preparation:

1. Process all ingredients through a juicer.
2. Stir the juice well to combine.
3. Serve immediately or refrigerate for up to 24 hours.

How to Use: To aid with liver cleansing, have one glass of beet juice every day, ideally first thing in the morning when you're not hungry.

Drink with Ginger and Turmeric Liver Flush

Intended Use: helps to increase the mechanisms involved in liver detoxification and reduce inflammation.

Ingredients:

- 1 tsp turmeric powder
- ½ tsp ginger powder
- Juice of 1 lemon
- 1 cup warm water
- 1 tsp olive oil

Preparation:

1. In a mug, combine turmeric, ginger, and lemon juice.

2. Add warm water and stir well to combine all ingredients.
3. Stir in olive oil for added detoxification benefits.

How to Use: For seven days in a row, drink this flush drink first thing in the morning on an empty stomach to help with liver cleaning. Take a week off, then try again if needed.

Green Detox Smoothie

Intended Use: provides a high-nutrient blend to support liver function and overall detoxification.

Ingredients:

- 1 cup fresh spinach
- ½ cup cilantro
- 1 green apple, cored and sliced
- ½ cucumber, sliced
- Juice of 1 lemon
- 1 tbsp chia seeds
- 1 cup water or coconut water

Preparation:

1. Combine all ingredients in a blender.
2. Blend on high until smooth.
3. If the smoothie is too thick, add more water or coconut water until desired consistency is reached.

How to Use: Drink this smoothie every day, ideally first thing in the morning, to help your body begin its natural cleansing process.

Dandelion Detox Tea

Intended Use: has inherent diuretic qualities that aid in renal function and liver cleansing.

Ingredients:

- 2 tbsp dried dandelion leaves
- 4 cups boiling water
- Lemon slice and honey (optional)

Preparation:

1. Place dandelion leaves in a large teapot.
2. Pour boiling water over the leaves and let steep for 10 minutes.
3. Strain the tea into cups.
4. Add a slice of lemon and honey to taste if desired.

How to Use: To assist in the cleansing of the liver and kidneys, drink one to two cups every morning.

Tea Made with Milk Thistle Seeds

Intended Use: Supports liver health and regeneration with the protective properties of milk thistle.

Ingredients:

- 1 tbsp milk thistle seeds
- 2 cups water

Preparation:

1. Crush the milk thistle seeds with a mortar and pestle to release their active compounds.
2. Boil water in a pot and add the crushed seeds.
3. Simmer for 20 minutes.
4. Strain the tea into a mug.

How to Use: Take one cup of milk thistle tea every day to safeguard and enhance the health of your liver.

Avocado and Kale Salad for Liver Health

Intended Use: A salad that is high in antioxidants, healthy fats, and fiber to help with liver function and detoxification.

Ingredients:

- 2 cups chopped kale
- 1 ripe avocado, diced
- ½ cup walnuts, chopped
- ¼ cup cranberries
- Dressing: 2 tbsp apple cider vinegar,

- 1 tbsp lemon juice,
- 1 tbsp extra-virgin olive oil, salt, and pepper

Preparation:

1. Combine kale, avocado, walnuts, and cranberries in a large salad dish.
2. In a small bowl, whisk together apple cider vinegar, lemon juice, olive oil, salt, and pepper to create the dressing.
3. Drizzle the dressing over the salad and toss gently to combine.

How to Use: Incorporate this salad into your meals 2-3 times a week for liver health and detoxification support.

Herbal Supplements for Liver Support

Intended Use: offers a practical means of consuming herbs that are recognized for their ability to help the liver.

Ingredients:

- Dried burdock root powder
- Dried dandelion root powder
- Dried milk thistle seed powder
- Empty capsules

Preparation:

1. In a bowl, mix equal parts of burdock root, dandelion root, and milk thistle seed powders.
2. Using a small spoon or a capsule machine, fill empty capsules with the herbal powder mixture.
3. Close the capsules.

How to Use: For optimal liver health and cleansing, take one or two capsules twice a day, ideally with meals, along with water.

Lemon Water's detoxifying properties

Intended Use: Lemon's alkalizing properties stimulate liver function and help the body eliminate toxins.

Ingredients:

- Juice of 1 lemon
- 1 cup warm water

Preparation:

1. Squeeze the juice of one lemon into a cup of warm water.
2. Stir to mix well.

How to Use: Drink lemon water first thing in the morning daily to support liver health and promote detoxification.

Spread of Cilantro Pesto Detox

Intended Use: This pesto is perfect for assisting liver detoxification because cilantro is well-known for its strong metal detoxifying qualities.

Ingredients:

- 2 cups fresh cilantro leaves
- ½ cup almonds or pine nuts
- 2 cloves garlic
- ½ cup extra-virgin olive oil
- Juice of 1 lemon
- Salt to taste

Preparation:

1. In a food processor, combine cilantro, nuts, and garlic. Pulse until finely chopped.
2. With the processor running, slowly add olive oil and lemon juice until well combined.
3. Season with salt to taste.

How to Use: To help with liver health and detoxification, spread this cilantro pesto over whole-grain bread or stir it into pasta meals on a daily basis.

Liver tonic with apple cider vinegar

Intended Use: Apple cider vinegar supports liver function and aids in detoxification by balancing blood pH levels.

Ingredients:

- 2 tbsp organic apple cider vinegar (with the "mother")
- 1 cup water

- Honey to taste (optional)

Preparation:

1. Mix apple cider vinegar with water in a glass.
2. Add honey to taste if desired.

How to Use: Take this tonic every day, preferably in the morning or right before meals, to promote liver cleansing and facilitate digestion.

IMPROVED IMMUNE DEFENSE

Elderberry Syrup to Boost Immunity

Intended Use: increases immunity and has antiviral qualities with elderberries, which are very antioxidant-rich.

Ingredients:

- 1 cup dried elderberries
- 4 cups water
- 1 cinnamon stick
- 1 tsp dried ginger root
- 1 cup raw honey

Preparation:

1. Combine elderberries, water, cinnamon stick, and dried ginger in asaucepan.
2. Bring to a boil, reduce heat, and simmer for about 45 minutes to anhour until the liquid has reduced by half.
3. Remove from heat, cool, and strain into a bowl.
4. Add raw honey to the liquid and stir until well combined.
5. Store the syrup in a sealed glass bottle in the refrigerator.

How to Use: For immune support, use 1 tbsp daily; if you have the flu or cold, take it every 3–4 hours. Due to honey, it is not advised for infants under one year old.

Turmeric and Black Pepper Tea

Intended Use: strengthens the immune system and lowers inflammation thanks to the potent mix of black pepper and turmeric.

Ingredients:

- 1 tsp turmeric powder
- ¼ tsp black pepper
- 1 tbsp lemon juice
- 1 tsp honey
- 1 cup hot water

Preparation:

1. In a mug, combine turmeric powder and black pepper.
2. Add hot water and stir well to dissolve the turmeric.
3. Mix in lemon juice and honey for taste.
4. Stir well and sip slowly.

How to Use: Drink this tea once daily, especially during cold and flu season,to enhance immune defense.

Ginger and Garlic Broth to Boost Immunity

Intended Use: Garlic and ginger, which are both recognized for their antibacterial and anti-inflammatory qualities, boost the immune system.

Ingredients:

- 4 cups vegetable broth
- 4 cloves garlic, minced
- 1 inch ginger root, sliced
- ½ onion, chopped
- Optional: Carrots, celery, and other vegetables for added nutrients

Preparation:

1. In a large pot, combine vegetable broth, garlic, ginger, and onion.Add any other vegetables as desired.
2. Bring to a boil, then reduce heat and simmer for 20-30 minutes.
3. Strain the broth, discarding solids.
4. Serve the broth warm.

How to Use: Pour a cup or two of this soup into your diet each day to help strengthen your immune system.

Berry and Spinach Smoothie

Intended Use: provides an abundance of minerals, vitamins, and antioxidants to boost immunity.

Ingredients:

- 1 cup fresh spinach

- ½ cup mixed berries (blueberries, strawberries, raspberries)
- 1 banana
- 1 tbsp chia seeds
- 1 cup almond milk or water

Preparation:

1. Add spinach, mixed berries, banana, chia seeds, and almond milk orwater to a blender.
2. Blend until smooth.
3. Adjust consistency with more liquid if necessary.
4. Serve immediately to preserve nutrients.

How to Use: Drink one smoothie daily as a nutrient-rich snack or breakfastto boost the immune system.

Herbal Tea with Lemon Balm

Intended Use: Lemon balm, which has antiviral and mood-enhancing qualities, lowers stress and boosts immunological function.

Ingredients:

- 1 tbsp dried lemon balm leaves
- 1 cup boiling water

Preparation:

1. Place lemon balm leaves in a tea infuser or directly in a mug.
2. Pour boiling water over the leaves.
3. Cover and let steep for 10 minutes.
4. Strain and enjoy the tea warm.

How to Use: Drink 1-2 cups of lemon balm tea daily to support immunehealth and reduce stress.

Carrot and Sweet Potato Soup

Intended Use: provides vitamin A and C from carrots and sweet potatoes to support immunological wellness.

Ingredients:

- 2 sweet potatoes, peeled and cubed
- 4 carrots, peeled and sliced
- 1 onion, diced
- 4 cups vegetable broth
- 1 tsp turmeric
- Salt and pepper to taste
- 1 tbsp olive oil

Preparation:

1. In a large pot, heat olive oil over medium heat. Add onions and cook until translucent.
2. Add sweet potatoes, carrots, turmeric, and vegetable broth.
3. Bring to a boil, then reduce heat and simmer until vegetables aretender.
4. Puree the soup with an immersion blender or in batches in a blender.
5. Season with salt and pepper to taste.

How to Use: Warm up this hearty dish to boost your immunity, particularly in the winter months when colds and flu are common.

Rich in Probiotics Sauerkraut

Intended Use: The probiotic-rich homemade sauerkraut improves immunity and digestive health.

Ingredients:

- 1 medium cabbage, shredded
- 1 tbsp sea salt

Preparation:

1. In a large bowl, mix the shredded cabbage with sea salt. Massage thesalt into the cabbage until it starts to release water.
2. Pack the cabbage tightly into a clean jar, pressing down until thewater rises above the cabbage.
3. Cover the jar with a cloth and secure with a rubber band.
4. Let it ferment at room temperature for 3-10 days, checking daily toensure the cabbage is submerged in brine.

5. Once fermented, seal the jar and store in the refrigerator.

How to Use: Every day, add a tiny amount of sauerkraut to your meals to improve your immune system and digestion.

Pumpkin Seed Pesto with Zinc.

Intended Use: Zinc from pumpkin seeds, which is essential for preserving a healthy immune system, improves immunological function.

Ingredients:

- 1 cup pumpkin seeds, toasted
- 2 cups fresh basil leaves
- 2 cloves garlic
- ½ cup olive oil
- Juice of 1 lemon
- Salt and pepper to taste

Preparation:

1. In a food processor, combine pumpkin seeds, basil leaves, and garlic.
2. Gradually add olive oil and lemon juice until the mixture becomes asmooth paste.
3. Season with salt and pepper.
4. Store in an airtight container in the refrigerator.

How to Use: To get extra zinc into your diet, use this pesto as a dip, spread, or sauce for pasta and salads.

Anti-Immune Berry Compote

Intended Use: delivers a tasty berry compote along with a substantial dose of antioxidants and vitamin C.

Ingredients:

- 2 cups mixed frozen berries
- 2 tbsp water
- 1 tbsp honey or maple syrup
- Zest of 1 orange

Preparation:

1. In a saucepan over medium heat, combine berries, water, honey ormaple syrup, and orange zest.
2. Cook until the berries are soft and the sauce has thickened, about 10 minutes.
3. Let cool before serving.

How to Use: Enjoy this compote over yogurt, oatmeal, or pancakes for adelicious way to boost your immune system.

Kefir Smoothie for Healthy Immune System and Gut

Intended Use: uses kefir's probiotics to improve intestinal health and boost immunity generally.

Ingredients:

- 1 cup kefir
- 1 banana
- ½ cup frozen blueberries
- 1 tbsp flaxseed meal
- Honey to taste

Preparation:

1. Combine kefir, banana, blueberries, and flaxseed meal in a blender.
2. Blend until smooth.
3. Sweeten with honey to taste.
4. Serve immediately.

How to Use: Regularly consume this smoothie—especially in the morning—to boost your immune system and promote healthy digestion.

MOOD STABILIZATION

Tea Using Holy Basil (Tulsi) to Promote Emotional Balance

Intended Use: Holy basil's adaptogenic qualities help to stabilize mood and lower stress.

Ingredients:

- 1 tbsp dried holy basil leaves
- 1 cup boiling water
- Honey or lemon (optional)

Preparation:

1. Place holy basil leaves in a cup or tea infuser.
2. Pour boiling water over the leaves and cover the cup.
3. Steep for 5-10 minutes.
4. Strain the tea and add honey or lemon if desired.

How to Use: Sip one to two cups each day to help with stress relief and mood stability.

Powdered Ashwagandha Root Tonic

Intended Use: uses ashwagandha root's adaptogenic properties to lower anxiety and regulate mood.

Ingredients:

- ½ tsp Ashwagandha root powder
- 1 cup warm milk (dairy or plant-based)
- Honey to taste

Preparation:

1. Mix Ashwagandha powder into warm milk until fully dissolved.
2. Add honey to sweeten if desired.
3. Drink before bedtime.

How to Use: Drink every night to help balance your mood and minimize stress.

Capsules with Adaptogenic Herbal Blend

Intended Use: gives a daily dosage of adaptogens to support mood stabilization and the control of the body's stress response.

Ingredients:

- Equal parts powdered Ashwagandha, Rhodiola, and Holy Basil
- Empty capsules

Preparation:

1. Mix the powdered herbs together thoroughly.
2. Fill empty capsules with the herb blend using a capsule machine.
3. Store in a cool, dry place.

How to Use: To help stabilize your mood throughout the day, take one or two capsules first thing in the morning with some water.

Smoothie High in Omega-3 for Brain Health

Intended Use: increases the stabilization of mood by consuming omega-3 fatty acids, which are essential for brain function.

Ingredients:

- 1 banana
- 1 cup spinach
- ¼ cup walnuts
- 2 tbsp ground flaxseeds
- 1 cup almond milk
- Ice cubes (optional)

Preparation:

1. Combine all ingredients in a blender.
2. Blend until smooth.
3. Serve immediately for maximum freshness.

How to Use: Drink this smoothie first thing in the morning to get mood-stabilizing nutrients to start your day.

Relaxing Tea Blend with Chamomile and Lavender

Intended Use: uses the relaxing qualities of chamomile and lavender to promote relaxation and mood stability.

Ingredients:

- 1 tsp dried lavender flowers
- 1 tsp dried chamomile flowers
- 1 cup boiling water

Preparation:

1. Mix lavender and chamomile flowers in a tea infuser or teapot.
2. Pour boiling water over the flowers and steep for 5-7 minutes.
3. Strain and serve warm.

How to Use: Drink in the evening to unwind and promote a balanced mood.

Mood Lifting Oil with Rosemary and Lemon Balm

Intended Use: elevates the spirit and eases tension with the calming aroma of rosemary and lemon balm.

Ingredients:

- 10 drops lemon balm essential oil
- 10 drops rosemary essential oil
- 2 tbsp carrier oil (such as almond or jojoba oil)

Preparation:

1. Mix lemon balm and rosemary essential oils with the carrier oil in asmall bottle.
2. Shake well to combine.

How to Use: When feeling anxious or in need of a mood boost, apply to wrists or temples. After use, exercise caution when exposed to direct sunlight, especially if the oil contains citrus.

Maca Powder with Chocolate Mood Drink

Intended Use: Enhances mood and vitality with the mood-boosting qualities of cacao and the natural energizing qualities of maca powder.

Ingredients:

- 1 tbsp maca powder
- 1 tbsp cacao powder
- 1 banana
- 1 cup almond milk
- Ice cubes

Preparation:

1. Place all ingredients in a blender.
2. Blend until smooth.
3. Serve immediately.

How to Use: Enjoy this smoothie as a midday pick-me-up to stabilize moodand boost energy.

Nut-Rich, Vitamin-Rich Trail Mix

Intended Use: enhances brain health and mood stability with a blend of nuts and seeds high in B vitamins.

Ingredients:

- ¼ cup almonds
- ¼ cup walnuts
- ¼ cup sunflower seeds
- ¼ cup pumpkin seeds
- A pinch of sea salt

Preparation:

1. Combine all nuts and seeds in a bowl and toss with sea salt.
2. Store in an airtight container for freshness.

How to Use: Throughout the day, munch on this trail mix to keep your energy up and your mood steady.

Saffron Mood-Stable Tincture

Intended Use: Saffron's mood-boosting qualities improve mood and promote emotional well-being.

Ingredients:

- A pinch of saffron threads
- 1 cup boiling water
- Honey to taste

Preparation:

1. Steep saffron threads in boiling water for 10 minutes.
2. Strain the water into a cup, discarding the saffron threads.
3. Add honey to taste and stir well.

How to Use: Take one capsule each day, ideally first thing in the morning, to help stabilize your mood.

Ginkgo Biloba Tea for Mood and Memory

Intended Use: Supports cognitive function and mood stabilization withGinkgo Biloba.

Ingredients:

- 1 tsp dried Ginkgo Biloba leaves
- 1 cup boiling water

Preparation:

1. Steep Ginkgo Biloba leaves in boiling water for 10 minutes.
2. Strain and drink warm.

How to Use: To improve emotional stability and cognitive performance, have one cup every morning.

HEALTHY SKIN

Antioxidant Green Tea Face Tone

Intended Use: green tea gives the skin antioxidants and reduces irritation.

Ingredients:

- 1 cup brewed green tea (strong)
- 1 tsp apple cider vinegar
- 5 drops tea tree oil

Preparation:

1. Brew green tea and allow it to cool.
2. Mix in apple cider vinegar and tea tree oil.
3. Pour the mixture into a clean bottle.

How to Use: Apply to the face with a cotton ball after cleansing, morningand evening.

Avocado Moisturizer

Intended Use: Avocado's natural lipids and vitamins nourish and moisturize skin.

Ingredients:

- ½ ripe avocado
- 1 tbsp honey
- 1 tsp yogurt (optional for extra hydration)

Preparation:

1. Mash the avocado in a bowl until smooth.
2. Mix in honey and yogurt until well combined.
3. Apply to clean face and leave on for 15-20 minutes.
4. Rinse off with warm water.

How to Use: For optimal skin hydration and nutrition, use once a week.

Healing Salve with Calendula and Chamomile

Intended Use: Calendula and chamomile have natural anti-inflammatory qualities that soothe and cure injured or irritated skin.

Ingredients:

- ¼ cup calendula petals
- ¼ cup chamomile flowers
- ½ cup coconut oil
- ¼ cup beeswax pellets
- 10 drops lavender essential oil

Preparation:

1. Gently melt coconut oil in a double boiler, then add calendula petals and chamomile flowers. Simmer on low heat for 2-3 hours to infuse the oil.
2. Strain the oil through a cheesecloth to remove the petals and flowers.
3. Return the infused oil to the double boiler, add beeswax pellets, andmelt together.
4. Remove from heat and stir in lavender essential oil.
5. Pour into small jars or tins and let cool until solid.

How to Use: Apply twice daily or as needed to clean skin in areas of irritation, dryness, or small cuts.

Soothing Bath Soak with Oatmeal

Intended Use: Oatmeal soothes dry, irritated skin and acts as a mild exfoliant.

Ingredients:

- 1 cup colloidal oatmeal (finely ground oats)
- ¼ cup baking soda
- 5 drops chamomile essential oil

Preparation:

1. Mix colloidal oatmeal and baking soda in a bowl.
2. Stir in chamomile essential oil.
3. Add the mixture to a warm bath and stir to distribute.

How to Use: To calm and moisturize the skin, soak in the tub for ten to fifteen minutes. Use as required or once a week.

Herbal Hair Rinse: Strength and Shine

Intended Use: uses natural herbs to increase luster and strengthen hair.

Ingredients:

- 2 tbsp dried nettle leaves
- 2 tbsp dried rosemary leaves
- 1 quart boiling water

Preparation:

1. Place nettle and rosemary in a large bowl.
2. Pour boiling water over the herbs and let steep for 1 hour.
3. Strain the liquid and let cool.

How to Use: Use as a final rinse after shampooing. Do not rinse out. Useregularly for best results.

Aloe Vera Gel for Cooling

Intended Use: Aloe vera soothes and moisturizes burnt or irritated skin.

Ingredients:

- ½ cup aloe vera gel
- 10 drops peppermint essential oil
- 5 drops lavender essential oil

Preparation:

1. Mix aloe vera gel with peppermint and lavender essential oils in abowl.
2. Transfer to a clean jar or bottle.
3. Store in the refrigerator for extra cooling effect.

How to Use: Apply as necessary to afflicted areas to provide cooling relief. Wonderful for sunburn or following sun exposure.

Rosewater Hydrating Mist

Intended Use: The calming effects of rosewater hydrate and revitalize skin.

Ingredients:

- 1 cup rosewater
- 1 tbsp glycerin
- 5 drops rose essential oil

Preparation:

1. Combine rosewater, glycerin, and rose essential oil in a clean spraybottle.
2. Shake well to mix.

How to Use: For hydration and refreshment, spritz on the face and neck as required throughout the day.

Brightening Face Scrub with Turmeric

Intended Use: Brightens and evens out skin tone with the anti-inflammatory and antioxidant properties of turmeric.

Ingredients:

- 2 tbsp ground turmeric
- ¼ cup fine sugar
- ¼ cup coconut oil

Preparation:

1. Mix turmeric and sugar in a bowl.
2. Stir in coconut oil until a paste forms.
3. Gently massage onto wet skin in circular motions, avoiding the eyearea.
4. Rinse off with warm water and pat dry.

How to Use: Use 1-2 times per week to enhance complexion and brighten skin.

Sea Salt Hair Scrub

Intended Use: Sea salt exfoliates the scalp, eliminating dead skin cells and encouraging the development of healthy hair.

Ingredients:

- 2 tbsp sea salt
- 2 tbsp olive oil
- 5 drops rosemary essential oil

Preparation:

1. Mix sea salt, olive oil, and rosemary essential oil in a bowl.
2. Apply to damp scalp in sections, gently massaging in circularmotions.
3. Rinse thoroughly and follow with shampoo.

How to Use: Use as needed or once a month to revitalize the scalp and encourage hair growth.

Yogurt and Cucumber Calming Face Mask

Intended Use: Soothes and hydrates the skin with the cooling effects ofcucumber and the moisturizing properties of yogurt.

Ingredients:

- ½ cucumber, pureed
- 2 tbsp plain yogurt

Preparation:

1. Mix cucumber puree and yogurt until well combined.
2. Apply to clean face and leave on for 15-20 minutes.
3. Rinse off with cool water.

How to Use: Use once or twice a week to soothe inflamed skin and provide soothing moisture.

IMPROVING THE QUALITY OF SLEEP

Chamomile and Lavender Sleeping Tea

Intended Use: uses the relaxing qualities of lavender and chamomile to encourage relaxation and enhance the quality of sleep.

Ingredients:

- 2 tbsp dried chamomile flowers
- 1 tbsp dried lavender buds
- 2 cups boiling water
- Honey (optional)

Preparation:

1. Combine chamomile and lavender in a teapot.
2. Pour boiling water over the herbs and cover.
3. Steep for 10 minutes.
4. Strain into cups and add honey to taste, if desired.

How to Use To encourage a good night's sleep, have a drink thirty minutes before going to bed.

Valerian Root Sleep Tincture

Intended Use: Valerian root's calming properties promote sleep and lessen nocturnal awakenings.

Ingredients:

- ¼ cup dried valerian root
- 1 cup vodka or apple cider vinegar (for alcohol-free version)
- Glass jar with lid

Preparation:

1. Place valerian root in the glass jar.
2. Pour vodka or vinegar over the root, ensuring it's completelycovered.
3. Seal the jar and store in a cool, dark place for 4-6 weeks, shakingdaily.
4. Strain the tincture into a clean bottle.

How to Use: Take 20-30 drops in water 30 minutes before bedtime.

Pillow Spray for Better Sleep

Intended Use: uses the calming aroma of essential oils to create a peaceful sleeping atmosphere.

Ingredients:

- 1 cup distilled water
- 4 drops lavender essential oil
- 2 drops chamomile essential oil
- 2 drops sweet orange essential oil
- Spray bottle

Preparation:

1. Add essential oils to the spray bottle.
2. Fill the bottle with distilled water.
3. Shake well to mix.

How to Use: Before you go to bed, spritz your pillow and the surrounding area in your bedroom.

Blended Ashwagandha Sleep Aid

Intended Use: includes ashwagandha, an adaptogen with a reputation for lowering stress and encouraging sound sleep.

Ingredients:

- 1 tsp ashwagandha powder
- 1 banana
- 1 cup spinach
- 1 tbsp almond butter
- 1 cup almond milk
- 1 tsp honey (optional)

Preparation:

1. Place all ingredients in a blender.
2. Blend until smooth.

3. Serve immediately.

How to Use: To reap the benefits of this smoothie's sleep-promoting qualities, have it in the evening, a few hours before going to bed.

Rich in Magnesium Banana Smoothie

Intended Use: magnesium, which is well-known for promoting relaxation and improving sleep, helps support sleep.

Ingredients:

1. 1 ripe banana
2. 1 cup spinach
3. 1 tbsp almond butter
4. 1 cup almond milk
5. A pinch of cinnamon

Preparation:

- Place all ingredients in a blender.
- Blend until smooth.
- Serve immediately.

How to Use: Take one hour before going to bed to enhance the quality of your sleep.

Passionflower Herbal Sleeping Capsules

Intended Use: uses the relaxing properties of passionflower to lessen anxiety and lengthen sleep.

Ingredients:

- Dried passionflower
- Empty capsules
- Capsule machine (optional)

Preparation:

1. Grind dried passionflower into a fine powder.
2. Use a capsule machine or a small spoon to fill empty capsules withthe powder.
3. Close the capsules.

How to Use: Take one or two capsules an hour before going to bed.

Hops and Lemon Balm Sleep Aid Tea

Intended Use: combines hops and lemon balm to help induce deep sleep and lessen insomnia.

Ingredients:

- 1 tbsp dried lemon balm leaves
- 1 tsp dried hops
- 2 cups boiling water

Preparation:

1. Place lemon balm and hops in a teapot.
2. Pour boiling water over the herbs.
3. Steep for 10 minutes, then strain.
4. Drink warm.

How to Use: Take 30 minutes before bed to improve the quality of your sleep.

Cedarwood Foot Rub Oil

Intended Use: The calming aroma of cedarwood eases physical tension and gets the mind ready for sleep.

Ingredients:

- 2 tbsp carrier oil (such as almond or jojoba)
- 6 drops cedarwood essential oil

Preparation:

1. Mix the carrier oil and cedarwood essential oil in a small bowl.
2. Transfer to a bottle for storage.

How to Use: Massage a small amount onto your feet before bedtime to aidrelaxation and sleep.

Warm Milk Drink with Nutmeg

Intended Use: Utilizes the natural sedative properties of nutmeg to improvesleep quality.

Ingredients:

- 1 cup milk (dairy or plant-based)
- ¼ tsp ground nutmeg
- Honey to taste (optional)

Preparation:

1. Gently heat the milk in a saucepan.
2. Stir in ground nutmeg.
3. Add honey to taste, if using.
4. Pour into a cup and drink warm.

How to Use: To promote a restful night's sleep, have a drink before going to bed.

Jasmine Flower Bath Soak for Bedtime

Intended Use: The calming aroma of jasmine blossoms relaxes the body and clears the mind.

Ingredients::

- ¼ cup dried jasmine flowers
- 1 cup Epsom salt
- 5 drops lavender essential oil

Preparation:

1. Mix jasmine flowers, Epsom salt, and lavender essential oil in abowl.
2. Add to a warm bath and stir to dissolve.

How to Use: Take advantage of this bath soak an hour before going to bed to ensure a peaceful sleep.

REDUCTION OF STRESS AND FATIGUE

Ginseng Energy Boost Tea

Intended Use: Enhances energy levels and reduces fatigue with the naturalstimulating properties of ginseng.

Ingredients::

- 1 inch fresh ginseng root, thinly sliced (or 1 tsp ginseng powder)
- 2 cups boiling water
- Lemon slice and honey to taste

Preparation:

1. Place ginseng slices (or powder) in a teapot.
2. Pour boiling water over ginseng and steep for 5-10 minutes.
3. Strain the tea into a cup, add lemon and honey to taste.

How to Use: Drink in the morning or early afternoon to help fight weariness and increase energy.

Salts for Relaxation in Lavender Bath

Intended Use: a calming combination of lavender and Epsom salts that encourages relaxation and lowers tension.

Ingredients::

- 1 cup Epsom salts
- ½ cup baking soda
- 10 drops lavender essential oil
- Dried lavender flowers (optional)

Preparation:

1. In a bowl, mix Epsom salts and baking soda.
2. Add lavender essential oil (and dried flowers if using) and mix well.
3. Store in an airtight jar.

How to Use: To warm bath water, add ¼ to ½ cup of bath salts. For at least twenty minutes, soak to relieve tension and exhaustion.

Tonic with Adaptogen Ashwagandha

Intended Use: uses ashwagandha, an adaptogen well renowned for its ability to reduce stress, to support general vitality while lowering tiredness and stress.

Ingredients::

- 1 tsp ashwagandha powder
- 1 cup warm milk (dairy or plant-based)
- Honey to taste
- A pinch of cinnamon (optional)

Preparation:

1. Warm the milk in a saucepan over low heat.
2. Stir in the ashwagandha powder until fully dissolved.
3. Remove from heat and add honey and cinnamon to taste.
4. Pour into a mug and enjoy warm.

How to Use: Drink once a day, ideally in the evening, to assist decompress and ease weariness and tension.

Rose Rhodiola Morning Elixir

Intended Use: increases energy and stress tolerance with Rhodiola Rosea, an adaptogen that has been shown to have anti-fatigue properties.

Ingredients::

- 1 tsp Rhodiola Rosea powder
- 1 cup hot water
- Juice of ½ lemon
- Honey to taste

Preparation:

1. Dissolve Rhodiola Rosea powder in hot water.
2. Add lemon juice and honey, stirring until well combined.
3. Drink warm.

How to Use: Take one capsule in the morning to help you feel less stressed and tired all day.

Tea with Holy Basil (Tulsi) to Reduce Stress

Intended Use: holy basil, often known as tulsi, has relaxing effects that help reduce tension and anxiety.

Ingredients::

- 2 tbsp dried holy basil leaves
- 2 cups boiling water
- Honey or lemon to taste

Preparation:

1. Steep holy basil leaves in boiling water for 10 minutes.
2. Strain and add honey or lemon to taste.
3. Serve warm or chilled.

How to Use: Drink 1-2 cups daily to help manage stress levels and promoterelaxation.

The Power Smoothie Adaptogen

Intended Use: uses a combination of nutrient-rich nutrients and adaptogenic herbs to reduce stress and increase energy.

Ingredients::

- 1 cup spinach
- 1 banana
- ½ cup blueberries
- 1 tbsp almond butter
- 1 tsp maca powder
- 1 tsp ashwagandha powder
- 1 cup almond milk

Preparation:

1. Place all ingredients in a blender.
2. Blend on high until smooth.
3. Serve immediately.

How to Use: Have this smoothie first thing in the morning or before to doing anything that demands stamina and resistance to stress.

Energy Bars with Chia Seeds

Intended Use: Provides sustained energy and reduces fatigue with nutrient-rich chia seeds, nuts, and dried fruit.

Ingredients::

- 1 cup oats
- ½ cup chia seeds
- ½ cup almonds, chopped
- ½ cup dried cranberries
- ¼ cup honey
- ¼ cup almond butter

Preparation:

1. Mix oats, chia seeds, almonds, and cranberries in a bowl.
2. Heat honey and almond butter in a saucepan until melted. Pour overdry ingredients and stir to combine.
3. Press the mixture into a lined baking dish and refrigerate until set.
4. Cut into bars.

How to Use: For an energy boost and stress relief on hectic days, eat a bar as needed.

Blend of Peppermint and Rosemary Focus Diffuser

Intended Use: enhances focus and lessens mental tiredness with a stimulating peppermint and rosemary aroma.

Ingredients::

- 5 drops peppermint essential oil
- 5 drops rosemary essential oil
- Water for diffuser

Preparation:

1. Fill the diffuser with water in accordance with the manufacturer's recommendations.
2. Add peppermint and rosemary essential oils.

3. Turn on the diffuser and enjoy the aroma.

How to Use: Use to improve attention and lessen mental tiredness during work or study periods.

Stress-Relieving Citrus and Sage Spray

Intended Use: With the grounding properties of sage and the uplifting aroma of citrus, this blend uplifts and refreshes the soul while lowering stress.

Ingredients::

- ½ cup distilled water
- ½ cup witch hazel
- 10 drops orange essential oil
- 5 drops lemon essential oil
- 5 drops sage essential oil

Preparation:

1. Combine water and witch hazel in a spray bottle.
2. Add essential oils and shake well to blend.
3. Label the bottle for future reference.

How to Use: Spritz all around your intimate area for a quick fix on stress reduction. Steer clear of direct skin and eye contact.

Nighttime Tea with Chamomile and Lemon Balm

Intended Use: uses chamomile and lemon balm to reduce tension and exhaustion while encouraging relaxation and sound sleep.

Ingredients::

- 1 tbsp dried lemon balm
- 1 tbsp dried chamomile flowers
- 2 cups boiling water

Preparation:

1. Place lemon balm and chamomile in a teapot.
2. Pour boiling water over the herbs and steep for 10 minutes.
3. Strain and serve warm.

How to Use: Thirty minutes before going to bed, have a drink to help you relax, reduce tension, and be ready for a pleasant sleep.

VISION ASSISTANCE

Smoothie to Improve Vision Using Blueberries and Spinach

Intended Use: uses the antioxidants in blueberries and the vitamin A in spinach to support eye health and vision.

Ingredients::

- 1 cup fresh blueberries
- 1 cup fresh spinach
- 1 banana
- 1 cup almond milk
- 1 tbsp flaxseed

Preparation:

1. Place blueberries, spinach, banana, almond milk, and flaxseed into ablender.
2. Blend until smooth.
3. Serve immediately for the best flavor and nutrient retention.

How to Use: To maintain good eye health and general eyesight, drink this smoothie every day, ideally in the morning.

Bilberry Herbal Tea

Intended Use: enhanced night vision and lessens ocular tiredness with bilberry, an antioxidant-rich fruit.

Ingredients::

- 1 tsp dried bilberry
- 1 cup boiling water
- Honey (optional)

Preparation:

1. Steep bilberry in boiling water for 10 minutes.
2. Strain the tea into a cup.
3. Add honey to taste, if desired.

How to Use: To promote good vision, sip on 1-2 cups of bilberry tea every day, particularly in the evening.

Rich in Omega-3 Chia Seed Pudding

Intended Use: chia seeds' rich omega-3 concentration supports eye health.

Ingredients::

- 3 tbsp chia seeds
- 1 cup coconut milk
- 1 tbsp maple syrup
- ½ tsp vanilla extract
- Fresh berries for topping

Preparation:

1. In a bowl, mix chia seeds, coconut milk, maple syrup, and vanillaextract.
2. Cover and refrigerate overnight or for at least 4 hours.
3. Serve topped with fresh berries.

How to Use: Consume this pudding for breakfast or as a snack two or three times a week to get omega-3 fatty acids that will support vision.

Turmeric and Carrot Eye Health Drink

Intended Use: uses turmeric's anti-inflammatory qualities and beta-carotene from carrots to improve eyesight support.

Ingredients::

- 4 large carrots, peeled
- 1 inch of fresh turmeric root
- 1 apple, cored
- ½ lemon, peeled

Preparation:

1. Juice the carrots, turmeric root, apple, and lemon using a juicer.
2. Stir the juice well before serving.
3. Drink immediately or store in a glass jar in the refrigerator for up to24 hours.

How to Use: Consume one glass of this juice daily to benefit from its vision-supporting nutrients.

Veggie and Walnut Salad

Intended Use: Provides essential nutrients for eye health, including luteinfrom kale and omega-3 fatty acids from walnuts.

Ingredients::

- 2 cups chopped kale
- ½ cup chopped walnuts
- 1 avocado, diced
- ¼ cup dried cranberries
- Dressing: olive oil, lemon juice, salt, and pepper

Preparation:

1. Combine kale, walnuts, avocado, and dried cranberries in a largesalad bowl.
2. In a small bowl, whisk together olive oil, lemon juice, salt, andpepper to taste.
3. Pour dressing over the salad and toss well to combine.

How to Use: Consume this salad frequently, ideally two or three times per week, to optimize the advantages of eyesight support.

Green Tea and Citrus Antioxidant Drink

Intended Use: Protects eyes from oxidative stress and supports overall visionhealth with antioxidants from green tea and vitamin C from citrus.

Ingredients::

- 1 green tea bag
- 1 cup hot water
- Juice of ½ lemon
- 1 tsp honey (optional)
- A few slices of orange (for garnish)

Preparation:

1. Steep green tea bag in hot water for 3-5 minutes.
2. Remove the tea bag and add lemon juice and honey, stirring untildissolved.
3. Garnish with orange slices.

4. Serve hot or chilled.

How to Use: Every day, especially in the morning, sip this antioxidant-rich tea to promote eye health and guard against vision-related problems.

Pumpkin Seed Snack High in Zinc

Intended Use: zinc supports eye health, which is important for preserving the health of the retina.

Ingredients::

- 1 cup pumpkin seeds
- 1 tbsp olive oil
- Sea salt to taste

Preparation:

1. Preheat the oven to 300°F (150°C).
2. Toss pumpkin seeds with olive oil and sea salt.
3. Spread on a baking sheet and roast for 15-20 minutes, stirringoccasionally.
4. Let cool before serving.

How to Use: Snack on these pumpkin seeds throughout the day or sprinklethem on salads and soups to boost your zinc intake.

Goji Berry and Almond Trail Mix

Intended Use: uses vitamin E from almonds and the antioxidants in goji berries to improve the health of your eyes.

Ingredients::

- ½ cup goji berries
- 1 cup almonds
- ½ cup sunflower seeds
- ¼ cup dark chocolate chips

Preparation:

1. Combine goji berries, almonds, sunflower seeds, and dark chocolatechips in a bowl.
2. Mix well and store in an airtight container.

How to Use: Every day, have a tiny handful of this trail mix as a nutritious snack to help maintain eye health.

Ginger and Sweet Potato Soup

Intended Use: provides anti-inflammatory properties from ginger and vitamin A from sweet potatoes to support eyesight.

Ingredients::

- 2 large sweet potatoes, peeled and cubed
- 1 inch of ginger, grated
- 1 onion, chopped
- 4 cups vegetable broth
- Salt and pepper to taste
- Coconut cream (optional for garnish)

Preparation:

1. Sauté onion and ginger in a large pot until softened.
2. Add sweet potatoes and vegetable broth. Bring to a boil, then simmeruntil sweet potatoes are tender.
3. Blend the soup until smooth using an immersion blender.
4. Season with salt and pepper. Serve hot, garnished with coconutcream if desired.

How to Use: Enjoy the vision-supporting elements of this soup many times a week, especially during the colder months.

Rice with Saffron Vision Support

Intended Use: uses saffron's vision-improving qualities to enhance clarity of vision and maintain eye health.

Ingredients::

- 1 cup basmati rice, rinsed
- 2 cups water
- A pinch of saffron threads
- 1 tbsp olive oil
- Salt to taste

Preparation:

1. Soak saffron threads in ¼ cup warm water for 10 minutes.
2. In a pot, bring 2 cups water to a boil. Add olive oil, salt, and saffronwater.
3. Add rice and return to a boil. Reduce heat, cover, and simmer untilrice is tender and liquid is absorbed.
4. Fluff with a fork before serving.

How to Use: To get the benefits of this saffron rice's vision-supporting qualities, include it in your meals two or three times each week.

SUPPORT FOR WEIGHT LOSS

Apple Cider Vinegar Breakfast Drink

Intended Use: Supports weight loss and improves digestion with thedetoxifying effects of apple cider vinegar.

Ingredients:

- 2 tbsp apple cider vinegar (with the mother)
- 1 cup warm water
- 1 tbsp honey (optional)
- A pinch of cayenne pepper (optional)

Preparation:

1. Mix apple cider vinegar in warm water.
2. If preferred, add the cayenne pepper and honey, and whisk until thoroughly mixed.
3. Drink on an empty stomach in the morning.

How to Use: Pour one cup in the morning every day to aid with detoxification and weight reduction.

Cinnamon and Honey Weight Loss Tea

Intended Use: uses honey and cinnamon to help control blood sugar levels and promote weight reduction.

Ingredients:

- 1 tsp ground cinnamon
- 1 cup boiling water
- 1 tsp honey

Preparation:

1. Add cinnamon to boiling water and let it steep for 15 minutes.
2. Strain the mixture and stir in honey until dissolved.
3. Drink warm.

How to Use: Take one serving each day, ideally in the morning to aid with weight reduction.

Green Tea Booster for Metabolism

Intended Use: increases metabolism and facilitates fat burning thanks to green tea's natural qualities.

Ingredients:

- 1 green tea bag or 1 tsp loose green tea leaves
- 1 cup boiling water
- Juice of ½ lemon
- 1 tsp grated ginger

Preparation:

1. Steep green tea and grated ginger in boiling water for 3-5 minutes.
2. Remove tea bag or strain loose leaves.
3. Stir in lemon juice.
4. Drink warm or chilled.

How to Use: Drink two to three cups per day, preferably before meals, to increase metabolism and promote weight reduction.

Hot Ginger Lemonade

Intended Use: Ginger and lemon stimulate digestion and increase metabolism.

Ingredients:

- 2 inches of fresh ginger root, grated
- Juice of 2 lemons
- 4 cups water
- Honey to taste
- A pinch of cayenne pepper

Preparation:

1. Boil water and add grated ginger. Simmer for 10 minutes.
2. Strain ginger and let the water cool to room temperature.
3. Add lemon juice, honey, and cayenne pepper. Stir well.
4. Serve chilled or at room temperature.

How to Use: Drink 1-2 glasses daily, especially before meals, to enhancedigestion and metabolism.

Fennel Tea with Seeds

Intended Use: Fennel seeds aid with digestion and minimize bloating.

Ingredients:

- 1 tsp fennel seeds
- 1 cup boiling water

Preparation:

1. Crush the fennel seeds slightly to release their oils.
2. Steep in boiling water for 10 minutes.
3. Strain and drink warm.

How to Use: After meals, consume to help weight reduction and improve digestion.

Grapefruit and Avocado Salad

Intended Use: Encourages weight loss with the healthy fats in avocado andthe fat-burning properties of grapefruit.

Ingredients:

- 1 ripe avocado, sliced
- 1 grapefruit, sectioned
- Mixed salad greens
- Dressing: olive oil, white wine vinegar, salt, and pepper

Preparation:

1. Arrange mixed salad greens on a plate.
2. Top with sliced avocado and grapefruit sections.
3. Whisk together olive oil, vinegar, salt, and pepper for the dressing.
4. Drizzle dressing over the salad just before serving.

How to Use: Savor this salad as a light and refreshing lunch to aid with weight loss.

Pineapple and Spirulina Smoothie

Intended Use: increases metabolism and aids in weight reduction thanks to pineapple's high-protein spirulina and bromelain content.

Ingredients:

- 1 tsp spirulina powder
- 1 cup fresh pineapple chunks
- 1 banana
- 1 cup spinach
- 1 cup coconut water

Preparation:

1. Place all ingredients in a blender.
2. Blend until smooth.
3. Serve immediately.

How to Use: Smoothie in the morning to boost metabolism and aid in weight reduction.

Carrot and Beet Salad: A Detoxification

Intended Use: nutrient-dense beets and carrots aid in weight reduction and cleansing.

Ingredients:

- 2 medium beets, grated
- 2 carrots, grated
- 2 tbsp olive oil
- 1 tbsp lemon juice
- Salt and pepper to taste
- Fresh parsley, chopped

Preparation:

1. Combine grated beets and carrots in a bowl.
2. In a separate bowl, whisk together olive oil, lemon juice, salt, andpepper.
3. Pour dressing over the beet and carrot mixture and toss to coatevenly.
4. Garnish with chopped parsley.

How to Use: To help with detoxification and weight reduction, eat this salad as a light dinner or as a side dish.

Berry and Chia Seed Pudding

Intended Use: offers a nutrient-dense, high-fiber meal or snack to aid with weight loss.

Ingredients:

- ¼ cup chia seeds
- 1 cup almond milk
- ½ cup mixed berries
- 1 tbsp honey or maple syrup

Preparation:

1. Mix chia seeds with almond milk and let sit for at least 30 minutes orovernight in the fridge, stirring occasionally.
2. Once set, top with mixed berries and sweeten with honey or maplesyrup.

How to Use: Eat this for breakfast or as a snack to help you stay full and lose weight.

Juice of Kale, Apple, and Lemon for Cleaning

Intended Use: helps with weight reduction and cleansing with a drink that's high in nutrients.

Ingredients:

- 2 cups kale leaves
- 1 green apple, cored
- Juice of 1 lemon
- 1 inch ginger root
- 1 cucumber

Preparation:

1. Wash all produce thoroughly.
2. Juice kale, apple, lemon, ginger, and cucumber in a juicer.
3. Stir the juice well and drink immediately.

How to Use: Drink this juice first thing in the morning on an empty stomach to aid with weight reduction and cleansing.

MENTAL SPEED AND DIRECTION

Blend of Peppermint and Rosemary Focus Oil

Intended Use: increases concentration and mental clarity thanks to the energizing effects of peppermint and rosemary essential oils.

Ingredients:

- 10 drops rosemary essential oil
- 10 drops peppermint essential oil
- 30 ml carrier oil (such as almond or jojoba oil)

Preparation:

1. In a small bottle, mix the rosemary and peppermint essential oils withthe carrier oil.
2. Shake well to combine.
3. Label the bottle for future reference.

How to Use: For improved mental clarity and attention, apply a tiny quantity to the back of the neck and temples. Because essential oils are strong, use them carefully.

Supercharged Smoothie Bowl

Intended Use: Provides essential nutrients for brain health and cognitivefunction, including omega-3 fatty acids, antioxidants, and vitamins.

Ingredients:

- 1 banana
- ½ cup blueberries
- 1 tbsp chia seeds
- 1 tbsp flaxseeds
- 1 cup spinach
- 1 cup almond milk
- Toppings: sliced almonds, additional blueberries, coconut flakes

Preparation:

1. Process the banana, blueberries, spinach, chia seeds, flax seeds, and almond milk

until smooth.
2. Pour into a bowl and add toppings as desired.

How to Use: Savor this smoothie bowl for breakfast to give you a steady supply of energy and mental clarity throughout the day.

Trail Mix with Pumpkin and Walnut Seeds for Brain Health

Intended Use: Omega-3-rich walnuts and magnesium-rich pumpkin seeds, which are essential for cognitive function, support brain health.

Ingredients:

- ½ cup walnuts
- ½ cup pumpkin seeds
- ¼ cup dark chocolate chips
- ¼ cup dried cranberries

Preparation:

1. Combine walnuts, pumpkin seeds, dark chocolate chips, and driedcranberries in a bowl.
2. Mix well and store in an airtight container.

How to Use: Throughout the day, munch on this trail mix to keep your brain fueled and improve concentration and mental clarity.

Almond Butter and Chocolate Energy Balls

Intended Use: Boosts mental energy and focus with the antioxidant-richcacao and healthy fats in almond butter.

Ingredients:

- 1 cup oats
- ½ cup almond butter
- ¼ cup cacao powder
- ¼ cup honey or maple syrup
- A pinch of salt

Preparation:

1. Mix oats, almond butter, cacao powder, honey, and salt in a bowluntil well

combined.
2. Roll the mixture into small balls.
3. Place the balls on a baking sheet and refrigerate for at least 30minutes to set.

How to Use: To keep your concentration and mental energy up throughout the day, munch on these energy balls.

Ginkgo Biloba and Green Tea Brain BoostDrink

Intended Use: When combined with the antioxidant properties of green tea, ginkgo biloba supports cognitive function and improves blood flow to the brain.

Ingredients:

- 1 tsp dried Ginkgo Biloba leaves
- 1 green tea bag
- 1 cup boiling water
- Honey or lemon to taste (optional)

Preparation:

1. Steep Ginkgo Biloba leaves and the green tea bag in boiling water for5 minutes.
2. Remove the tea bag and strain out Ginkgo Biloba leaves.
3. Add honey or lemon to taste if desired.

How to Use: Every day, have one cup in the morning or early afternoon to help with attention and mental clarity.

Clarity Tea with Herbs

Intended Use: lowers mental tiredness and improves attention with a combination of brain-boosting herbs.

Ingredients:

- 1 tsp dried rosemary
- 1 tsp dried peppermint
- 1 tsp dried gotu kola
- 2 cups boiling water

Preparation:

1. Mix the dried herbs together.

2. Steep the herbal blend in boiling water for 10 minutes.
3. Strain and serve the tea warm or chilled.

How to Use: To stay focused and have mental clarity throughout the day, make yourself a cup of this herbal tea in the morning and another in the early afternoon.

Lion's Mane Mushroom Soup

Intended Use: Known for its ability to improve cognition, Lion's Mane mushrooms support nerve growth factor and brain health.

Ingredients:

- 1 cup Lion's Mane mushrooms, chopped
- 1 onion, diced
- 2 cloves garlic, minced
- 4 cups vegetable broth
- 1 cup coconut milk
- Salt and pepper to taste
- Fresh herbs for garnish (parsley or thyme)

Preparation:

1. Sauté onion and garlic in a pot until translucent.
2. Add Lion's Mane mushrooms and cook for 5 minutes.
3. Pour in vegetable broth and bring to a simmer for 20 minutes.
4. Stir in coconut milk and season with salt and pepper.
5. Blend the soup until smooth if desired.
6. Garnish with fresh herbs before serving.

How to Use: Consume this soup regularly to benefit from the cognitive-enhancing effects of Lion's Mane mushrooms.

Rich in Omega-3 Flaxseed Oil Dressing

Intended Use: includes a large amount of omega-3 fatty acids in the diet to promote cognitive and mental wellness.

Ingredients:

- ¼ cup flaxseed oil

- 2 tbsp apple cider vinegar
- 1 tbsp lemon juice
- 1 tsp Dijon mustard
- Salt and pepper to taste

Preparation:

1. Whisk together flaxseed oil, apple cider vinegar, lemon juice, andDijon mustard in a bowl.
2. Season with salt and pepper.
3. Store in an airtight container in the refrigerator.

How to Use: To increase your consumption of omega-3 fatty acids for brain health, pour this dressing over cooked veggies or use it over salads.

Brain Power Breakfast with Avocado and Egg

Intended Use: offers a high concentration of choline, vitamin E, and omega-3 fatty acids, all of which are proven to promote cognitive performance and brain health.

Ingredients:

- 1 ripe avocado, halved and pitted
- 2 eggs
- Salt and pepper to taste
- Whole-grain toast for serving

Preparation:

1. Scoop out a little avocado flesh to create space for the egg.
2. Crack an egg into each avocado half.
3. Season with salt and pepper.
4. Bake at 425°F (220°C) for 15-20 minutes, until the egg is cooked toyour liking.
5. Serve with whole-grain toast.

How to Use: Savor this nutrient-dense breakfast to give your brain the best start to the day.

Avocado and Sardine Brain Health Toast

Intended Use: combines avocado's healthful fats with sardines' omega-3 fatty acids to create a snack that improves cognitive function.

Ingredients:

- 2 slices of whole-grain bread, toasted
- 1 ripe avocado, mashed
- 1 can of sardines in olive oil, drained
- Lemon juice to taste
- Salt and pepper to taste

Preparation:

1. Spread mashed avocado onto toasted bread slices.
2. Top each slice with sardines.
3. Season with lemon juice, salt, and pepper.

How to Use: Consume this nutrient-dense toast for breakfast or as a midday snack to enhance cognitive and mental clarity.

COLD AND FLU RELIEF

Ginger Turmeric Cold Relief Tea

Intended Use: This tea aims to soothe sore throats, reduce inflammation, and boost the immune system's antiviral properties.

Ingredients:

- 2 inches of fresh ginger root (thinly sliced)
- 1 tsp turmeric powder or 1-inch piece of fresh turmeric (sliced)
- 4 cups water
- Honey (to sweeten)
- Juice of 1 lemon

Preparation:

1. Boil ginger and turmeric in water, then simmer for 10-15 minutes.
2. Strain into a mug, add honey and lemon juice.
3. Stir well and drink warm.

How to Use: Drink 2-3 cups daily during cold or flu symptoms for relief and immunity boost.

Homemade Chicken Soup

Intended Use: Provides comfort and nutrients for cold and flu relief, including hydration and electrolytes.

Ingredients:

- 1 whole chicken or chicken parts (with bone)
- 2 liters water
- 1 onion (chopped)
- 2 carrots (chopped)
- 2 celery stalks (chopped)
- Salt and pepper (to taste)
- Fresh herbs like parsley or thyme (optional)

Preparation:

1. Boil chicken in water, then simmer with vegetables and herbs.
2. Shred chicken, discard bones, and serve hot.

How to Use: Enjoy 2-3 bowls daily when feeling unwell to stay hydrated and nourished.

Echinacea and Elderberry Immune Booster

Intended Use: This mixture aims to strengthen the immune system, aiding in the fight against cold and flu symptoms.

Ingredients:

- 1 tbsp dried echinacea
- 1 tbsp dried elderberries
- 4 cups water
- Honey and lemon juice (to taste)

Preparation:

1. Combine echinacea, elderberries, and water in a pot.
2. Boil, then let it simmer for 20 minutes.
3. Strain into a container, squeezing out the herb juices.
4. Add honey and lemon juice as desired.
5. Drink warm or refrigerate for up to a week.

How to Use: Consume 1 cup 2-3 times daily upon first signs of cold or flu symptoms. Continue until symptoms alleviate.

Peppermint and Eucalyptus Steam Inhalation

Intended Use: Clears congestion and soothes irritated nasal passages and throats.

Ingredients:

- 3 drops peppermint essential oil
- 3 drops eucalyptus essential oil
- Bowl of boiling water

Preparation:

1. Pour boiling water into a bowl.
2. Add peppermint and eucalyptus essential oils.
3. Lean over the bowl, covering head and bowl with a towel.

4. Inhale deeply for 5-10 minutes.

How to Use: Perform steam inhalation 1-2 times daily as needed for congestion relief during colds and flu.

Garlic and Honey Immune-Supporting Paste

Intended Use: Boosts immunity with garlic's antiviral properties and honey's soothing effects.

Ingredients:

- 3-4 cloves garlic, finely minced or crushed
- 2 tbsp honey

Preparation:

1. Combine minced garlic and honey in a bowl.
2. Mix thoroughly to form a paste.
3. Let sit for a few hours or overnight.

How to Use: Take ½ tsp of paste 2-3 times daily at the onset of cold or flu symptoms. Do not consume on an empty stomach.

Vitamin C-Packed Citrus Salad

Intended Use: Refreshing salad high in vitamin C to support the immune system and reduce cold and flu severity.

Ingredients:

- 2 oranges, peeled and sliced
- 1 grapefruit, peeled and sliced
- 1 tbsp chopped mint leaves
- Drizzle of honey (optional)

Preparation:

1. Arrange citrus slices on a plate.
2. Sprinkle with mint leaves and honey if desired.

How to Use: Enjoy as part of daily meals to boost vitamin C intake during cold and flu season.

Bone Broth

Intended Use: Nutrient-rich broth supports immune function and provides essential minerals for recovery.

Ingredients:

- 2 pounds mixed bones (beef, chicken, or fish)
- 2 carrots, roughly chopped
- 2 celery stalks, roughly chopped
- 1 onion, quartered
- 2 tbsp apple cider vinegar
- Herbs (optional)
- Water

Preparation:

1. Place bones in a pot, cover with water, add apple cider vinegar, and bring to a boil.
2. Reduce to a simmer, skim off foam, and add vegetables and herbs.
3. Simmer for 12-24 hours, adding water if needed.
4. Strain and store broth.

How to Use: Drink 1-2 cups warm daily to support immune health and recovery from cold and flu symptoms.

Hot Lemon and Honey Drink

Intended Use: Soothes sore throats, hydrates, and provides vitamin C for immune support.

Ingredients:

- Juice of 1 lemon
- 1 tbsp honey
- 1 cup hot water

Preparation:

1. Squeeze lemon juice into a mug.
2. Add honey and hot water.
3. Stir until honey dissolves.

How to Use: Drink as needed throughout the day to soothe a sore throat and stay hydrated.

Oregano Oil Capsules

Intended Use: Oregano oil's antimicrobial properties help fight cold and flu viruses.

Ingredients:

- Oregano essential oil
- Olive oil or coconut oil
- Empty capsules

Preparation:

1. Dilute oregano oil with olive or coconut oil.
2. Fill empty capsules with the oil mixture.

How to Use: Take one capsule twice daily with meals at first sign of cold or flu symptoms for up to 5 days. Consult a healthcare provider before use.

Thyme and Honey Cough Syrup

Intended Use: Eases coughing and soothes sore throats with thyme's expectorant properties and honey's soothing texture.

Ingredients:

- ¼ cup dried thyme
- 1 cup water
- 1 cup honey

Preparation:

1. Steep dried thyme in boiling water for 20 minutes.
2. Strain and heat thyme-infused water with honey.
3. Pour into a jar and let cool.

How to Use: Take 1 tsp as needed for cough relief and throat soothing. Refrigerate for up to a month.

ANXIETY REDUCTION

Tea Blend of Lavender and Chamomile

Intended Use: This blend of tea is intended to help those who are suffering anxiety by promoting relaxation, lowering stress levels, and calming the nervous system.

Ingredients:

- Two cups of boiling water
- One tbsp dried lavender flowers
- One tbsp dried chamomile flowers
- Honey (optional, for sweetness)

Preparation:

1. Combine lavender and chamomile in a teapot or infuser.
2. Pour boiling water over the herbs and cover.
3. Allow the tea to steep for 5-10 minutes, depending on desiredstrength.
4. Strain the tea into cups.
5. Sweeten with honey if preferred.

How to Use: When your worry starts to build up during the day, make a cup of this relaxing tea in the evening before going to bed. Frequent use can aid in stress management on a daily basis.

Ashwagandha Grounding Smoothie

Intended Use: Ashwagandha, which has adaptogenic qualities, is included in this smoothie to lower stress, regulate cortisol, and ease anxiety.

Ingredients:

- 1 tsp ashwagandha powder
- 1 banana
- ½ cup blueberries
- 1 cup spinach
- 1 cup almond milk
- A handful of almonds

Preparation:

1. Place all ingredients into a blender.
2. Blend on high until smooth and creamy.
3. Pour into a glass and enjoy immediately.

How to Use: Drink this smoothie in the morning to help you stay focused and stress-free, or in the evening to help you unwind and heal from a stressful day.

Capsules of Passionflower Herbal

Intended Use: Passionflower is well known for its ability to alleviate anxiety and enhance the quality of sleep. A practical approach to take passionflower for anxiety treatment is with these handmade capsules.

Ingredients:

- Dried passionflower powder
- Empty capsules

Preparation:

1. Purchase high-quality dried passionflower powder from a reputablesource.
2. Using a small spoon or a capsule machine, fill each empty capsulewith the powder.
3. Close the capsules according to the instructions.

How to Use: Take one capsule twice daily with water, especially during times of heightened anxiety or before bed to aid sleep.

Lemon Balm and Mint Stress Relief Water

Intended Use: A revitalizing herbal infusion of lemon balm and mint that helps reduce tension and anxiety while fostering a feeling of peace and wellbeing.

Ingredients:

- A handful of fresh lemon balm leaves
- A handful of fresh mint leaves
- 1 liter of water
- Ice cubes (optional)
- Slices of cucumber or lemon for added flavor (optional)

Preparation:

1. Rinse the lemon balm and mint leaves under cold water.
2. Bruise the leaves gently with your fingers to release their oils.
3. Fill a pitcher with water and add the bruised leaves.
4. Add ice cubes, cucumber, or lemon slices if using.
5. Refrigerate for at least an hour to allow the flavors to infuse.
6. Stir well before serving.

How to Use: In order to keep hydrated and lower anxiety, drink throughout the day. When taken before stressful situations or during times of high stress, it is extremely helpful.

Smoothie with Omega-3s to Reduce Anxiety

Intended Use: This smoothie contains omega-3 fatty acids from flaxseeds and walnuts, which are known to reduce anxiety and improve mood.

Ingredients:

- 1 banana
- ½ cup blueberries
- 1 tbsp ground flaxseeds
- 1 tbsp walnuts
- 1 cup spinach
- 1 cup almond milk

Preparation:

1. Place all ingredients in a blender.
2. Blend until smooth.
3. Pour into a glass and enjoy immediately.

How to Use: This smoothie may be had as a midday snack to sustain balanced energy and lowered anxiety levels throughout the day, or as a morning snack to get your day started with a mood boost.

Aromatherapy Stress Relief Roller

Intended Use: An aromatherapy roller combination including essential oils recognized for their relaxing characteristics, intended to alleviate anxiety and encourage relaxation while on the road.

Ingredients:

- 10 drops lavender essential oil
- 10 drops frankincense essential oil
- 5 drops bergamot essential oil
- Carrier oil (such as jojoba or almond oil)
- 10 ml roller bottle

Preparation:

1. Add essential oils to the roller bottle.
2. Fill the rest of the bottle with the carrier oil.
3. Cap the bottle and shake well to blend the oils.
4. Label the bottle for easy identification.

How to Use: Whenever you feel nervous, roll onto pressure points like the wrists, temples, and backs of the ears. To enhance the relaxing benefits, take deep breaths.

Nourishing Oatmeal Anxiety Relief Mask

Intended Use: A facial mask made with oatmeal and calming ingredients to soothe the skin and senses, reducing anxiety and encouraging relaxation.

Ingredients:

- ½ cup ground oatmeal
- 2 tbsp plain yogurt
- 1 tbsp honey
- A few drops of lavender essential oil

Preparation:

1. Mix ground oatmeal, yogurt, and honey in a bowl until a paste forms.
2. Add lavender essential oil and mix well.
3. Apply to clean, dry skin, leaving on for 15-20 minutes.
4. Rinse with warm water and pat dry.

How to Use: As part of a weekly self-care regimen, use this mask once to nourish the skin and soothe the mind.

Nighttime Valerian Root Tea

Intended Use: Valerian root tea is known for its sedative properties, which make it an excellent choice for relieving anxiety and promoting restful sleep.

Ingredients:

- 1 tsp dried valerian root
- 1 cup boiling water
- Honey or lemon to taste (optional)

Preparation:

1. Steep valerian root in boiling water for 10 minutes.
2. Strain the tea into a cup.
3. Add honey or lemon if desired.

How to Use: Thirty minutes before going to bed, have a cup of valerian root tea to reduce tension and enhance sleep.

Herbal Calming Bath Soak

Intended Use: A therapeutic bath soak that uses herbs and Epsom salts to relax the body, calm the mind, and relieve anxiety.

Ingredients:

- ½ cup Epsom salts
- ¼ cup dried lavender flowers
- ¼ cup dried rose petals
- A few drops of chamomile essential oil

Preparation:

1. Mix Epsom salts, lavender, and rose petals in a bowl.
2. Add chamomile essential oil and stir to combine.
3. Store in an airtight container.

How to Use: To heated bath water, add a good handful of the herbal bath soak. In order for the herbs and Epsom salts to do their calming effect, you should soak for at least 20 minutes.

Relieving Stress- Balm

Intended Use: A homemade balm made with essential oils and natural butters to relieve stress and anxiety, ideal for on-the-spot application.

Ingredients:

- 2 tbsp coconut oil
- 2 tbsp shea butter
- 10 drops lavender essential oil
- 5 drops frankincense essential oil
- 5 drops bergamot essential oil

Preparation:

1. Gently melt coconut oil and shea butter in a double boiler.
2. Remove from heat and let cool slightly.
3. Stir in essential oils.
4. Pour into a small container and let solidify.

How to Use: Apply on the back of the neck, the wrists, or the temples if you're feeling tense or nervous. Take a big breath after using.

BOOST ANTIOXIDANT

Detox Turmeric Ginger Brew

Intended Use: This brew combines turmeric and ginger, both known for their health benefits such as supporting liver function and enhancing the body's natural detoxification processes, to create an anti-inflammatory and antioxidant blend.

Ingredients:

- 1 tsp ground turmeric
- 1 tsp grated fresh ginger
- 2 cups boiling water
- Lemon slice and honey to taste

Preparation:

1. Add turmeric and ginger to boiling water in a pot.
2. Simmer for 10 minutes to allow the flavors and nutrients to infuse.
3. Strain the brew into a mug.
4. Add a slice of lemon and honey to enhance flavor and benefits.

How to Use: Before going to bed, sip on this tea in the evening to help with detoxification and digestion. It's especially helpful after indulging or when you feel like cleansing.

Mint Matcha Refreshment

Intended Use: This beverage combines matcha's high antioxidant content with mint's digestive aid for a refreshing and health-boosting drink, ideal for energy and focus without the jitters of coffee.

Ingredients:

- 1 tsp matcha green tea powder
- A handful of fresh mint leaves
- 2 cups hot water (not boiling)
- Honey (optional)

Preparation:

1. Whisk matcha powder in hot water until fully dissolved.

2. Bruise mint leaves and add them to the matcha mixture.
3. Let steep for 3-5 minutes.
4. Strain into a cup, adding honey if desired.

How to Use: To optimize your antioxidant intake and experience a natural energy boost that fosters alertness and overall well-being, drink in the morning or early afternoon.

Antioxidant Berry Citrus Tea

Intended Use: A potent blend designed to boost your body's defense against oxidative stress by combining the antioxidant power of berries with the vitamin C content of citrus. This tea is ideal for those looking to boost their immune system, protect their skin, and improve their overall vitality.

Ingredients:

- ½ cup mixed dried berries (blueberries, raspberries, strawberries)
- Peel of 1 organic orange (to ensure no pesticides)
- 2 cups boiling water
- Honey (optional, for sweetness)

Preparation:

1. Place mixed dried berries and orange peel in a tea infuser or directlyinto a teapot.
2. Pour boiling water over the ingredients and cover.
3. Steep for 5-7 minutes for full flavor and nutrient release.
4. Strain into a mug or pitcher.
5. Sweeten with honey if desired.

How to Use: Drink this tea first thing in the morning for a healthy antioxidant boost to your day, or as a revitalizing pick-me-up in the middle of the afternoon. Frequent consumption can promote cellular health and help fight free radicals.

Almond Sunset Rooibos Tea

Intended Use: This caffeine-free, antioxidant-rich tea combines the sweetness of rooibos with the nutty flavor of almonds, making it ideal for relaxing evenings while also providing an antioxidant boost.

Ingredients:

- 1 tbsp loose rooibos tea

- 1 tsp almond slices
- 2 cups boiling water
- Vanilla extract (a drop for flavor)

Preparation:

1. Combine rooibos tea and almond slices in a teapot.
2. Add boiling water and steep for 5-7 minutes.
3. Strain into mugs and stir in a drop of vanilla extract.

How to Use: Savor this calming tea in the evening to unwind and end your day with a rich, antioxidant-packed beverage.

Antioxidant Berry Smoothie

Intended Use: A nutrient-dense smoothie that combines the antioxidant power of mixed berries with the added benefits of chia seeds to improve cellular health, combat oxidative stress, and serve as a delicious, energizing snack or breakfast option.

Ingredients:

- ½ cup mixed frozen berries (blueberries, strawberries, raspberries)
- 1 tbsp chia seeds
- 1 cup almond milk (unsweetened)
- 1 banana for natural sweetness
- A handful of spinach for extra nutrients (optional)

Preparation:

1. Combine all ingredients in a blender.
2. Blend on high until smooth.
3. Adjust the consistency with more almond milk if needed.
4. Serve immediately for the best flavor and nutrient content.

How to Use: Have this smoothie as a mid-afternoon snack to naturally increase your energy levels and antioxidant consumption, or in the morning for a colorful start to your day.

Herbal Bath Soak Super Antioxidant

Intended Use: A relaxing bath soak infused with antioxidant-rich herbs like rosemary and green tea, designed to soothe the skin, relieve stress, and absorb antioxidants through the skin for an overall wellness boost.

Ingredients:

- ¼ cup dried rosemary leaves
- ¼ cup dried green tea leaves
- 1 cup Epsom salts
- A few drops of lavender essential oil for relaxation

Preparation:

1. Mix all the ingredients in a bowl.
2. Fill a bath with warm water and add the herbal mixture.
3. Soak in the bath for 20-30 minutes, allowing the skin to absorb the antioxidants.

How to Use: As part of your weekly self-care regimen, take this bath soak once to help lower stress, cleanse the body, and improve skin health by absorbing antioxidants.

Antioxidant Pudding with Walnut and Flaxseed

Intended Use: This pudding is not only delicious, but it is also high in omega-3 fatty acids, lignans, and antioxidants from walnuts and flaxseeds, all of which promote heart health and reduce inflammation.

Ingredients:

- 2 tbsp ground flaxseeds
- 1 tbsp crushed walnuts
- 1 cup coconut milk
- 1 tsp vanilla extract
- 1 tbsp maple syrup or to taste

Preparation:

1. Mix coconut milk, vanilla extract, and maple syrup in a bowl.
2. Stir in ground flaxseeds and let sit for 5 minutes to thicken.
3. Add crushed walnuts and mix well.
4. Refrigerate for at least an hour before serving.

How to Use: Serve as a satisfying snack or dessert. It's a fantastic method to add antioxidants to your diet, particularly for the advantages on heart health and inflammation reduction.

Apple Spice Cinnamon Immunity Tea

Intended Use: This warming tea combines the antioxidant benefits of apples and cinnamon with a spice blend to support immune health; it's ideal for cold weather or whenever you need a boost.

Ingredients:

- 1 organic apple, sliced thinly
- 1 cinnamon stick
- A pinch of ground cloves and nutmeg
- 2 cups boiling water
- Honey (optional)

Preparation:

1. Place apple slices, cinnamon stick, cloves, and nutmeg in a pot.
2. Cover with boiling water and simmer for 10-15 minutes.
3. Strain the mixture into mugs.
4. Sweeten with honey to taste.

How to Use: Drink to strengthen your immune system when the seasons change or whenever you want a warm, antioxidant-rich beverage.

Antioxidant Salad with Spinach and Avocado

Intended Use: This salad is a nutritional powerhouse, combining antioxidant-rich spinach with healthy fats from avocado. It aims to improve skin health, boost the immune system, and provide essential vitamins and minerals.

Ingredients:

- 2 cups fresh spinach leaves
- 1 ripe avocado, cubed
- ¼ cup sliced almonds
- ½ cup fresh blueberries
- Dressing: Olive oil, lemon juice, salt, and pepper to taste

Preparation:

1. Toss spinach leaves, avocado cubes, sliced almonds, and blueberriesin a large salad bowl.

2. Whisk together olive oil, lemon juice, salt, and pepper in a smallbowl.
3. Drizzle the dressing over the salad and toss gently to combine.

How to Use: Savor this salad as a light lunch or as an accompaniment to dinner. Its high antioxidant concentration promotes immune system and skin health in particular, as well as general wellness.

Anti-Aging, Antioxidant Face Mask

Intended Use: This face mask uses raw cocoa powder and honey's natural antioxidants to combat free radical damage, reduce aging signs, and provide a glowing complexion.

Ingredients:

- 2 tbsp raw cocoa powder (high in antioxidants)
- 1 tbsp raw honey (for its antibacterial and moisturizingproperties)
- 1 tsp cinnamon (optional, for enhanced blood flow)

Preparation:

1. Mix cocoa powder, honey, and cinnamon in a small bowl until youachieve a paste-like consistency.
2. Apply the mixture to clean, dry skin and leave on for 15-20 minutes.
3. Rinse off with warm water, gently pat dry, and follow up with your regular moisturizer.

How to Use: Once a week, use this mask to replenish your face, focusing on free radicals and encouraging a more youthful, glowing complexion.

ANTIOXIDANT DEFENSE ENHANCEMENT

Green Tea Blend and Pomegranate

Intended Use: A drink made by combining pomegranate's high antioxidant content with green tea's catechins to improve cellular and cardiovascular health.

Ingredients:

- ½ cup of fresh pomegranate seeds
- 1 tsp of green tea leaves
- 2 cups of water
- Honey (optional)

Preparation:

1. Steep green tea leaves in hot water for 3 minutes.
2. Blend pomegranate seeds with a splash of water, then strain to obtainthe juice.
3. Mix pomegranate juice with brewed green tea.
4. Sweeten with honey if desired.

How to Use: Drink one cup of this mix every day, ideally first thing in the morning, to help you meet your daily need of antioxidants. It is also a heart-healthy and refreshing option for a midday pick-me-up.

Capsules of Turmeric and Black Pepper

Intended Use: Turmeric powder capsules with a pinch of black pepper increase bioavailability, promoting anti-inflammatory and antioxidant benefits.

Ingredients:

- Turmeric powder
- Ground black pepper
- Empty capsules

Preparation:

1. Mix turmeric powder with a small amount of black pepper (ratio of 10:1).
2. Fill empty capsules with the mixture using a capsule machine or small spoon.

How to Use: Take one capsule daily, preferably with food, for maximum absorption. This program is especially helpful for people who want to strengthen their antioxidant and anti-inflammatory defenses.

Berry Compote Packed with Antioxidants

Intended Use: A versatile compote made from mixed berries that provides a delicious way to consume a variety of antioxidants via diet.

Ingredients:

- 2 cups mixed berries (blueberries, strawberries, raspberries)
- ¼ cup water
- 2 tbsp honey or maple syrup
- 1 tsp lemon juice

Preparation:

1. Combine all ingredients in a saucepan over medium heat.
2. Simmer until berries have softened and the mixture has thickened.
3. Cool and store in the refrigerator.

How to Use: For a tasty, nutrient-dense way to start the day, top yogurt, oats, or whole-grain pancakes with this compote. Enjoyed as a dessert, it provides a nutrient-rich and healthier alternative.

Cold infusion of Rosehip and Hibiscus.

Intended Use: A refreshing cold infusion that uses rosehip vitamin C and hibiscus anthocyanins to promote skin health and immune function.

Ingredients:

- 2 tbsp dried rosehip
- 2 tbsp dried hibiscus petals
- 1 liter of cold water
- Lemon slices and mint for flavor

Preparation:

1. Combine rosehip and hibiscus in a large jar filled with cold water.
2. Refrigerate overnight to allow flavors and nutrients to infuse.

3. Strain and serve with lemon and mint.

How to Use: Throughout the day, especially in the warmer months, sip this infusion to keep hydrated and provide your body with essential antioxidants. It's great for immune system support and skin health.

Juice from carrots and beets

Intended Use: A beverage high in beta-carotene from carrots and antioxidants from beets, intended to improve liver function and detoxification.

Ingredients:

- 2 large carrots
- 1 medium beetroot
- 1 apple for sweetness
- 1-inch piece of ginger

Preparation:

1. Juice all ingredients, stir well, and serve immediately.

How to Use: To optimize this juice's detoxifying properties, have a glass of it first thing in the morning on an empty stomach. It offers a plethora of antioxidants and is a lively method to boost liver function and your body's natural detoxification activities.

Herbal rinse with basil and lemon balm.

Intended Use: A herbal hair and skin rinse that protects and soothes with the antioxidants found in basil and lemon balm.

Ingredients:

- 1 tbsp dried basil leaves
- 1 tbsp dried lemon balm leaves
- 2 cups boiling water

Preparation:

1. Steep basil and lemon balm in boiling water for 20 minutes.
2. Strain and cool the infusion.
3. Use as a final rinse after showering.

How to Use: Pour this rinse carefully over your skin and hair as the last step in your shower regimen. If at all feasible, let it air dry to enhance the antioxidants' absorption. It can improve scalp health and calm the skin.

Avocado & Walnut Salad

Intended Use: A nutrient-dense salad high in antioxidants from avocado and walnuts that promotes heart health and reduces oxidative stress.

Ingredients:

- 1 ripe avocado, diced
- ½ cup walnuts, toasted and chopped
- Mixed greens
- Olive oil and balsamic vinegar for dressing

Preparation:

1. Toss avocado, walnuts, and mixed greens in a salad bowl.
2. Drizzle with olive oil and balsamic vinegar.

How to Use: At least three times a week, include this salad for lunch or supper to reap the benefits of the heart-healthy fats in avocado and the antioxidants in walnuts. This filling lunch fights oxidative stress and promotes cardiovascular health.

Face mask made with flaxseed and honey

Intended Use: A topical face mask made with flaxseed's omega-3 fatty acids and honey's antibacterial qualities to nourish skin and counteract oxidative damage.

Ingredients:

- 2 tbsp ground flaxseed
- 1 tbsp raw honey
- Water as needed

Preparation:

1. Mix flaxseed and honey, adding water until a paste forms.
2. Apply to clean skin, leave on for 15 minutes, then rinse.

How to Use: Once a week, use this mask on clean, dry skin. Because of its high antioxidant content, it is especially helpful for dry or aging skin, offering deep nutrition and defense against environmental stresses.

Ginger-Cinnamon Decoction

Intended Use: A warming decoction that stimulates digestion and increases antioxidant absorption by combining ginger and cinnamon.

Ingredients:

- 1-inch piece of fresh ginger, sliced
- 1 cinnamon stick
- 3 cups of water

Preparation:

1. Combine ginger, cinnamon, and water in a pot.
2. Bring to a boil, then simmer for 15 minutes.
3. Strain and enjoy warm or cold.

How to Use: Drink a cup of this warming infusion first thing in the morning to help your metabolism and digestion get going. Alternatively, savor it post-meal to improve nutritional absorption and digestion.

Spirulina with Pineapple Smoothie

Intended Use: A powerful smoothie that combines spirulina's antioxidants with pineapple's bromelain for digestive health and immune support.

Ingredients:

- 1 tsp spirulina powder
- 1 cup pineapple chunks
- 1 banana
- 1 cup spinach
- 1 cup coconut water

Preparation:

2. Blend all ingredients until smooth.

How to Use: Savor this smoothie in the morning or as a post-workout snack to help strengthen your immune system and restore your body. Spirulina and pineapple together provide a potent antioxidant dosage that supports healing and digestion.

STRESS REDUCTION

Stress Relief Water With Lemon Balm and Mint

Intended Use: A pleasant herbal water flavored with lemon balm and mint to reduce tension and anxiety while generating a sense of serenity and wellbeing.

Ingredients:

- A handful of fresh lemon balm leaves
- A handful of fresh mint leaves
- 1 liter of water
- Ice cubes (optional)
- Slices of cucumber or lemon for added flavor (optional)

Preparation:

3. Rinse the lemon balm and mint leaves under cold water.
4. Bruise the leaves gently with your fingers to release their oils.
5. Fill a pitcher with water and add the bruised leaves.
6. Add ice cubes, cucumber, or lemon slices if using.
7. Refrigerate for at least an hour to allow the flavors to infuse.
8. Stir well before serving.

How to Use: In order to keep hydrated and lower anxiety, drink throughout the day. When taken before stressful situations or during times of high stress, it is extremely helpful.

Smoothie with Grounding Ashwagandha

Intended Use: This smoothie contains ashwagandha, which is known for its adaptogenic effects, to help reduce stress, balance cortisol, and alleviate anxiety.

Ingredients:

- 1 tsp ashwagandha powder
- 1 banana
- ½ cup blueberries
- 1 cup spinach
- 1 cup almond milk

- A handful of almonds

Preparation:

1. Place all ingredients into a blender.
2. Blend on high until smooth and creamy.
3. Pour into a glass and enjoy immediately.

How to Use: Drink this smoothie in the morning to help you stay focused and stress-free, or in the evening to help you unwind and heal from a stressful day.

Blend of lavender and chamomile tea.

Intended Use: This tea blend is intended to calm the nervous system, relieve tension, and promote relaxation, making it beneficial for those suffering from anxiety.

Ingredients:

- 1 tbsp dried lavender flowers
- 1 tbsp dried chamomile flowers
- 2 cups boiling water
- Honey (optional, for sweetness)

Preparation:

9. Combine lavender and chamomile in a teapot or infuser.
10. Pour boiling water over the herbs and cover.
11. Allow the tea to steep for 5-10 minutes, depending on desiredstrength.
12. Strain the tea into cups.
13. Sweeten with honey if preferred.

How to Use: When your worry starts to build up during the day, make a cup of this relaxing tea in the evening before going to bed. Frequent use can aid in stress management on a daily basis.

Passion Flower Herbal Capsules

Intended Use: Passionflower is known for its ability to reduce anxiety and improve sleep quality. These handmade capsules provide an easy method to take passionflower for anxiety alleviation.

Ingredients:

- Dried passionflower powder
- Empty capsules

Preparation:

1. Purchase high-quality dried passionflower powder from a reputablesource.
2. Using a small spoon or a capsule machine, fill each empty capsulewith the powder.
3. Close the capsules according to the instructions.

How to Use: Take one capsule twice a day with water, preferably right before bed to help you fall asleep or during periods of increased worry.

Relaxing Herbal Bath Soak

Intended Use: A therapeutic bath soak that uses herbs and Epsom salts to relax the body, calm the mind, and relieve anxiety.

Ingredients:

- ½ cup Epsom salts
- ¼ cup dried lavender flowers
- ¼ cup dried rose petals
- A few drops of chamomile essential oil

Preparation:

1. Mix Epsom salts, lavender, and rose petals in a bowl.
2. Add chamomile essential oil and stir to combine.
3. Store in an airtight container.

How to Use: To heated bath water, add a good handful of the herbal bath soak. In order for the herbs and Epsom salts to do their calming effect, you should soak for at least 20 minutes.

Stress relief balm

Intended Use: A handcrafted balm created with essential oils and natural butters to ease stress and anxiety, ideal for on-the-spot application.

Ingredients:

- 2 tbsp coconut oil

- 2 tbsp shea butter
- 10 drops lavender essential oil
- 5 drops frankincense essential oil
- 5 drops bergamot essential oil

Preparation:

1. Gently melt coconut oil and shea butter in a double boiler.
2. Remove from heat and let cool slightly.
3. Stir in essential oils.
4. Pour into a small container and let solidify.

How to Use: Apply on the back of the neck, the wrists, or the temples if you're feeling tense or nervous. Take a big breath after using.

Nourishing oatmeal mask for anxiety relief.

Intended Use: A face mask made with oatmeal and relaxing substances to soothe the skin and senses, lowering anxiety and encouraging relaxation.

Ingredients:

- ½ cup ground oatmeal
- 2 tbsp plain yogurt
- 1 tbsp honey
- A few drops of lavender essential oil

Preparation:

1. Mix ground oatmeal, yogurt, and honey in a bowl until a paste forms.
2. Add lavender essential oil and mix well.
3. Apply to clean, dry skin, leaving on for 15-20 minutes.
4. Rinse with warm water and pat dry.

How to Use: As part of a weekly self-care regimen, use this mask once to nourish the skin and soothe the mind.

Aromatherapy Roller for Stress Relief

Intended Use: An aromatherapy roller combination including essential oils known for their relaxing effects, intended to alleviate anxiety and encourage relaxation while on the road.

Ingredients:

- 10 drops lavender essential oil
- 10 drops frankincense essential oil
- 5 drops bergamot essential oil
- Carrier oil (such as jojoba or almond oil)
- 10 ml roller bottle

Preparation:

1. Add essential oils to the roller bottle.
2. Fill the rest of the bottle with the carrier oil.
3. Cap the bottle and shake well to blend the oils.
4. Label the bottle for easy identification.

How to Use: Whenever you feel nervous, roll onto pressure points like the wrists, temples, and backs of the ears. To enhance the relaxing benefits, take deep breaths.

Valerian Root Nighttea

Intended Use: Valerian root tea is known for its calming properties, which make it an ideal choice for relieving anxiety and aiding peaceful sleep.

Ingredients:

- 1 tsp dried valerian root
- 1 cup boiling water
- Honey or lemon to taste (optional)

Preparation:

1. Steep valerian root in boiling water for 10 minutes.
2. Strain the tea into a cup.
3. Add honey or lemon if desired.

How to Use: Thirty minutes before going to bed, have a cup of valerian root tea to reduce tension and enhance sleep.

Anxiety-Reducing Smoothie with Omega-3

Intended Use: This smoothie contains omega-3 fatty acids from flaxseeds and walnuts, which are known to lower anxiety and boost mood.

Ingredients:

- 1 banana
- ½ cup blueberries
- 1 tbsp ground flaxseeds
- 1 tbsp walnuts
- 1 cup spinach
- 1 cup almond milk

Preparation:

1. Place all ingredients in a blender.
2. Blend until smooth.
3. Pour into a glass and enjoy immediately.

How to Use: This smoothie may be had as a midday snack to sustain balanced energy and lowered anxiety levels throughout the day, or as a morning snack to get your day started with a mood boost.

BONE HEALTH

Calcium-Rich Nettle Tea

Intended Use: Supports bone health by providing a high dose of plant-based calcium from nettle leaves, which is essential for maintaining strong bones and preventing osteoporosis.

Ingredients:

- 2 tbsp dried nettle leaves
- 1 liter of water

Preparation:

1. Boil water in a large pot.
2. Add dried nettle leaves to the boiling water and reduce heat.
3. Simmer for 10 minutes to extract the nutrients.
4. Strain the tea into a large pitcher or teapot.
5. Allow cooling slightly before serving.

How to Use: Have one or two cups per day. Nettle tea is a healthy approach to enhance bone density and general health, and it may be drunk warm or cold.

Bone-Building Broth

Intended Use: A nutrient-dense broth made from bones, rich in collagen,calcium, and magnesium, vital for bone health and density.

Ingredients:

- 2 pounds mixed bones (chicken, beef, or fish)
- 2 carrots, chopped
- 2 celery stalks, chopped
- 1 onion, quartered
- 1 tbsp apple cider vinegar
- Herbs (such as thyme or parsley)
- Water to cover

Preparation:

1. Place bones in a large stockpot and cover with water.

2. Add apple cider vinegar and let sit for 30 minutes (to help extractminerals from the bones).
3. Add vegetables and herbs to the pot.
4. Bring to a boil, then reduce heat and simmer, covered, for 12-24hours. Skim off any foam that rises.
5. Strain the broth, discarding solids.
6. Store in the refrigerator or freeze for later use.

How to Use: To maintain bone health and joint mobility, drink one cup of bone broth every day, either on its own or as a foundation for soups and stews.

Dandelion Greens Salad

Intended Use: Dandelion greens are high in calcium and vitamin K, bothessential for bone strength and prevention of bone loss.

Ingredients:

- 2 cups fresh dandelion greens, washed and chopped
- 1 avocado, diced
- ¼ cup sliced almonds
- Dressing: Olive oil, lemon juice, salt, and pepper

Preparation:

1. Toss dandelion greens and diced avocado in a salad bowl.
2. Top with sliced almonds.
3. In a small bowl, mix olive oil, lemon juice, salt, and pepper to create the dressing.
4. Drizzle the dressing over the salad and toss gently to combine.

How to Use: Eat this salad as a light dinner or as a side to increase your consumption of nutrients that promote healthy bones. Since dandelion greens are at their tenderest in the spring, it's very helpful during that season.

Sesame Seed Tahini Dressing

Intended Use: Enhances bone health with high levels of calcium and zincfound in sesame seeds, promoting bone repair and growth.

Ingredients:

- ¼ cup tahini (sesame seed paste)

- Juice of 1 lemon
- 2 tbsp olive oil
- 1 garlic clove, minced
- Salt and pepper to taste
- Water, as needed to thin the dressing

Preparation:

1. In a bowl, whisk together tahini, lemon juice, olive oil, and minced garlic until smooth.
2. Season with salt and pepper.
3. Add water a little at a time, whisking until desired consistency is achieved.

How to Use: Use as a dip or as a drizzle over salads to add extra nutrients that build bones to your diet. For optimal effects, enjoy frequently.

Magnesium-Rich Banana and Spinach Smoothie

Intended Use: Designed to provide a tasty, magnesium-rich treat thatsupports bone health, muscle function, and the body's calcium utilization.

Ingredients:

- 1 ripe banana
- 1 cup fresh spinach
- 1 tbsp chia seeds
- 1 cup almond milk
- A pinch of cinnamon (optional)

Preparation:

1. Place banana, spinach, chia seeds, and almond milk in a blender.
2. Blend on high until smooth.
3. Add a pinch of cinnamon for flavor and additional health benefits.

How to Use: To guarantee that you are getting enough magnesium for your bones and general health, have this smoothie in the morning or as a post-workout snack.

Herbal Horsetail Tea

Intended Use: Horsetail is a herb rich in silicon, a mineral crucial for bone regeneration and health. This tea aids in strengthening bones and improving their density.

Ingredients:

- 1 tsp dried horsetail
- 1 cup boiling water

Preparation:

1. Steep dried horsetail in boiling water for 10 minutes.
2. Strain the tea and allow it to cool slightly before drinking.

How to Use: Each day, sip one or two glasses of horsetail tea.It is highly advised for those who want to organically maintain the health of their bones.

Sardine and Kale Bone Health Salad

Intended Use: Sardines are rich in calcium and vitamin D, crucial for bone

health, while kale provides additional calcium and antioxidants. This salad isdesigned to offer a balanced meal that supports bone strength and density.

Ingredients:

- 1 can of sardines in olive oil, drained
- 2 cups of kale, chopped
- ½ avocado, sliced
- ¼ cup of cherry tomatoes, halved
- 1 tbsp lemon juice
- 1 tbsp extra virgin olive oil
- Salt and pepper to taste

Preparation:

1. In a large salad bowl, combine chopped kale, sliced avocado, andhalved cherry tomatoes.
2. In a small bowl, whisk together lemon juice, extra virgin olive oil,salt, and pepper to create the dressing.
3. Pour the dressing over the salad and toss to evenly coat.
4. Top the salad with sardines, breaking them into bite-sized pieces ifdesired.

How to Use: To get the most nutrients that promote healthy bones in your diet, serve this salad for a substantial lunch or dinner. It's perfect for people who want to improve their bone health organically through food. Savor this meal many times a week to get the benefits of its diverse variety of nutrients for maintaining bone health and general well-being.

Collard Greens and Garlic Sauté

Intended Use: Collard greens are an excellent source of calcium and vitaminK, essential for bone health. Garlic adds flavor and has been shown to have a positive effect on bone health.

Ingredients:

- 1 bunch collard greens, stems removed and leaves chopped
- 2 tbsp olive oil
- 2 cloves garlic, minced
- Salt and pepper to taste

Preparation:

1. Heat olive oil in a large skillet over medium heat.
2. Add minced garlic and sauté until fragrant, about 1 minute.
3. Add chopped collard greens, tossing to coat with oil and garlic.
4. Sauté until greens are wilted and tender, about 5-7 minutes.
5. Season with salt and pepper to taste.

How to Use: To maintain bone health and make sure you're getting enough of the essential elements that promote bone health, serve this sauté as a side dish to your meals two to three times a week.

Prune and Walnut Oatmeal

Intended Use: Prunes are known for their ability to improve bone densityand prevent bone loss, while walnuts add omega-3 fatty acids and antioxidants, supporting overall bone health.

Ingredients:

- ½ cup rolled oats
- 1 cup water or milk
- 5 prunes, chopped
- ¼ cup walnuts, chopped

- Honey or maple syrup to taste

Preparation:

1. Cook oats in water or milk according to package instructions.
2. Once cooked, stir in chopped prunes and walnuts.
3. Sweeten with honey or maple syrup as desired.

How to Use: Serve for breakfast several times a week to help maintain bone health. This is especially helpful for women who have gone through menopause and are worried about osteoporosis.

Almond and Fig Energy Balls

Intended Use: These energy balls are a delicious, nutrient-dense snack that provides calcium and magnesium from almonds and figs, vital for maintaining bone health and density.

Ingredients:

- 1 cup dried figs, stems removed
- 1 cup almonds
- 2 tbsp chia seeds
- 1 tbsp coconut oil
- A pinch of sea salt

Preparation:

1. In a food processor, blend almonds until they reach a coarse mealconsistency.
2. Add dried figs, chia seeds, coconut oil, and sea salt to the almondmeal in the food processor.
3. Blend until the mixture sticks together when pressed between fingers.
4. Take small portions of the mixture and roll into balls, about the sizeof a walnut.
5. Place the balls on a baking sheet lined with parchment paper andrefrigerate for at least an hour to set.

How to Use: In order to increase your intake of vital minerals for bone health, eat one or two energy balls as a snack in between meals. They're very helpful for recuperating from an exercise or for a rapid energy boost during the day.

BOOST IMMUNE SYSTEM

Honey and Garlic Immune Tonic

Intended Use: Due to the well-known antibacterial and antiviral qualities of garlic, this tonic is a great way to support the immune system.

Ingredients:

- 3-4 cloves of garlic, minced
- ½ cup raw honey

Preparation:

1. Combine minced garlic and honey in a jar, ensuring the garlic is fullycoated.
2. Seal the jar and let it sit for 3-5 days at room temperature.
3. Stir the mixture daily.

How to Use: To boost your immunity, take 1 tsp of this tonic first thing in the morning on an empty stomach.

Golden Milk with Turmeric

Intended Use: Curcumin, a substance found in turmeric, has potent anti-inflammatory and antioxidant properties that make it a great choice for immune support.

Ingredients:

- 1 cup almond milk or coconut milk
- 1 tsp turmeric powder
- ½ tsp cinnamon
- ¼ tsp ginger powder
- A pinch of black pepper (to enhance curcumin absorption)
- 1 tsp coconut oil
- Honey to taste

Preparation:

1. Heat the milk in a saucepan over medium heat.
2. Add turmeric, cinnamon, ginger, black pepper, and coconut oil.
3. Whisk the mixture well and heat until warm but not boiling.

4. Add honey to taste after removing from heat.

How to Use: Have a cup of golden milk every day, especially in the evening, to increase immunity and encourage rest.

Syrup of elderberries

Intended Use: Elderberry syrup is a powerful treatment with immune-boosting qualities that can help ward off and prevent colds and the flu.

Ingredients:

- ½ cup dried elderberries
- 2 cups water
- 1 cinnamon stick
- 5 cloves
- 1 piece of fresh ginger, about an inch long
- 1 cup raw honey

Preparation:

1. Combine elderberries, water, cinnamon, cloves, and ginger in asaucepan.
2. Bring to a boil, then reduce heat and simmer until the liquid isreduced by half, about 45 minutes.
3. Strain the mixture through a fine mesh strainer, pressing the berriesto extract all the juice.
4. Allow the liquid to cool to lukewarm, then stir in the raw honey untilwell combined.
5. Store in a glass bottle in the refrigerator.

How to Use: To increase immunity throughout the cold and flu season, take 1 tbsp daily. Take 1 tbsp every 3–4 hours until symptoms go away if you're already sick.

Pumpkin Seed Pesto with Zinc.

Intended Use: Zinc, which is necessary for healthy immune system function, is abundant in pumpkin seeds. A tasty way to get more zinc in your diet is with this pesto.

Ingredients:

- 1 cup pumpkin seeds, toasted
- 2 cups fresh basil leaves

- 2 cloves garlic
- ½ cup olive oil
- Salt and pepper to taste
- Juice of 1 lemon

Preparation:

1. In a food processor, combine pumpkin seeds, basil, and garlic.
2. Pulse while gradually adding olive oil until the mixture reaches your desired consistency.
3. Season with salt, pepper, and lemon juice to taste.

How to Use: Spread this pesto on toast, pour it into spaghetti, or use it as a vegetable dip to raise your intake of zinc from food and boost your immune system multiple times a week.

Tea with Lemon Ginger to Boost Immunity

Intended Use: This tea strengthens the immune system and eases sore throats by utilizing the inherent antiviral and antibacterial qualities of lemon and ginger.

Ingredients:

- 1-inch piece of fresh ginger, sliced
- Juice of ½ lemon
- 1 tsp raw honey
- 1 cup boiling water

Preparation:

1. Place ginger slices in a mug and pour boiling water over them.
2. Steep for 5 minutes, then remove the ginger.
3. Stir in lemon juice and raw honey until dissolved.

How to Use: Sip 1-2 cups daily to strengthen immunity and soothe sore throats, particularly during the cold and flu season.

Carrot and Sweet Potato Soup

Intended Use: Beta-carotene, a substance found in abundance in this soup, is a precursor to vitamin A, which is necessary for a strong immune system.

Ingredients:

- 2 large sweet potatoes, peeled and cubed
- 3 carrots, peeled and sliced
- 1 onion, chopped
- 4 cups vegetable broth
- 1 tsp ground turmeric
- Salt and pepper to taste
- 1 can coconut milk

Preparation:

1. In a large pot, sauté onion until translucent.
2. Add sweet potatoes, carrots, turmeric, and vegetable broth.
3. Bring to a boil, then simmer until vegetables are tender.
4. Blend the soup until smooth, either using an immersion blender or bytransferring to a blender.
5. Stir in coconut milk and season with salt and pepper.

How to Use: Serve warm, and eat a bowl every day, particularly in the winter or when you need a pick-me-up.

Berry and Spinach Smoothie

Intended Use: A superfood smoothie full of antioxidants, vitamins C and E, and other immune-supporting minerals from fresh berries and greens.

Ingredients:

- 1 cup fresh spinach
- ½ cup mixed berries (strawberries, blueberries, raspberries)
- 1 banana
- 1 cup almond milk
- 1 tbsp chia seeds

Preparation:

1. Combine all ingredients in a blender.
2. Blend on high until smooth.
3. Adjust the consistency with more almond milk if needed.

How to Use: For a healthy snack or breakfast, try this smoothie to boost your immune system every day.

Rich in Probiotics Sauerkraut

Intended Use: Sauerkraut and other fermented foods improve gut health, which is essential for a robust immune system.

Ingredients:

- 1 medium cabbage, finely shredded
- 1 tbsp sea salt

Preparation:

1. In a large bowl, mix the cabbage with sea salt, massaging the saltinto the cabbage until it starts to release liquid.
2. Pack the cabbage tightly into a clean jar, pressing down until theliquid rises above the cabbage.
3. Seal the jar loosely and let it sit at room temperature for 3-10 days,checking daily to ensure the cabbage is submerged.
4. Once fermented, store in the refrigerator.

How to Use: Consume a tiny amount of sauerkraut every day along with your meals to help your immune system and digestion.

Throat Spray with Oregano Oil

Intended Use: Because of the strong antibacterial qualities of oregano oil, this throat spray is a useful treatment for sore throats and early symptoms of disease.

Ingredients:

- 1 tbsp oregano oil
- ¼ cup distilled water
- 1 tsp sea salt

Preparation:

1. Dilute oregano oil in distilled water and add sea salt.
2. Pour the mixture into a small spray bottle.
3. Shake well before each use.

How to Use: When irritation in the throat appears, or if you've been exposed to sickness, spray straight against the back of your throat two to three times a day.

Chia Seed Pudding with Almond Milk

Intended Use: A dessert that boosts immunity and lowers inflammation, thanks to the omega-3 fatty acids from chia seeds.

Ingredients:

- ¼ cup chia seeds
- 1 cup unsweetened almond milk
- ½ tsp vanilla extract
- 2 tbsp maple syrup
- Fresh berries for topping

Preparation:

1. In a bowl, whisk together chia seeds, almond milk, vanilla extract,and maple syrup.
2. Cover and refrigerate for at least 4 hours, or overnight, until itachieves a pudding-like consistency.
3. Serve topped with fresh berries.

How to Use: Savor this pudding as a nutritious dessert or as a snack to increase your consumption of important fats and strengthen your immune system.

COLD AND FLU RELIEF

Elderberries and Echinacea as Immune Boosters

Intended Use: strengthens the immune system to aid in the more efficient reversal of cold and flu symptoms.

Ingredients:

- 1 tbsp dried echinacea
- 1 tbsp dried elderberries
- 4 cups water
- Honey and lemon juice to taste

Preparation:

1. Combine echinacea and elderberries with water in a pot.
2. Bring to a boil, then simmer for 20 minutes.
3. Strain the mixture into a container, squeezing the herbs to extracttheir juice.
4. Add honey and lemon juice to taste.
5. Drink warm or store in the refrigerator for up to a week.

How to Use: After the first hint of a cold or the flu, drink one cup two to three times a day. Drink till the symptoms go away.

Personalized Chicken Soup

Intended Use: supplies nutrition and comfort for the treatment of colds and the flu, including electrolytes and hydration.

Ingredients:

- 1 whole chicken or chicken parts (with bone)
- 2 liters of water
- 1 onion, chopped
- 2 carrots, chopped
- 2 celery stalks, chopped
- Salt and pepper to taste
- Fresh herbs like parsley or thyme (optional)

Preparation:

1. Place the chicken in a large pot and cover with water.
2. Bring to a boil, then reduce heat to simmer. Skim off any foam thatrises.
3. Add chopped vegetables and herbs. Season with salt and pepper.
4. Cover and simmer for 1-2 hours, or until the chicken is cooked
5. through.
6. Remove the chicken, shred the meat, and return it to the pot. Discardthe bones.
7. Adjust seasoning if necessary and serve hot.

How to Use: When feeling under the weather, have a bowl of this soup two or three times a day to keep fed and hydrated.

Inhalation of Peppermint and Eucalyptus Steam

Intended Use: reduces congestion and calms sore throats and nasal passages.

Ingredients:

- 3 drops peppermint essential oil
- 3 drops eucalyptus essential oil
- A bowl of boiling water

Preparation:

1. Carefully pour boiling water into a heat-proof bowl.
2. Add drops of peppermint and eucalyptus essential oils to the water.
3. Lean over the bowl and cover your head and the bowl with a towel totrap the steam.
4. Breathe deeply for 5-10 minutes.

How to Use: Inhale steam. For cold and flu treatment, use 1-2 times daily as required.

Tea with Ginger and Turmeric for Cold Relief

Intended Use: has antiviral qualities that soothe sore throats, lower inflammation, and strengthen the immune system.

Ingredients:

- 2 inches of fresh ginger root, thinly sliced
- 1 tsp turmeric powder or a 1-inch piece of fresh turmeric, sliced
- 4 cups of water

- Honey to sweeten
- Juice of 1 lemon

Preparation:

1. Add ginger and turmeric to water in a pot.
2. Bring to a boil, then simmer for 10-15 minutes.
3. Strain the tea into a mug, add honey to taste, and squeeze in thelemon juice.
4. Stir well and drink warm.

How to Use: Drink 2-3 cups daily when experiencing cold or flu symptomsfor relief and to boost immunity.

Hot Lemon and Honey Drink

Intended Use: Hydrates, soothes sore throats, and supplies vitamin C to boost immunity.

Ingredients:

- Juice of 1 lemon
- 1 tbsp honey
- 1 cup hot water

Preparation:

1. Squeeze the juice of one lemon into a mug.
2. Add honey.
3. Pour hot water into the mug and stir until the honey dissolvescompletely.
4. Drink while warm.

How to Use: Stay hydrated and ease sore throats by drinking as much as necessary throughout the day.

Bone Broth

Intended Use: Rich in nutrients, bone broth boosts immunity and supplies vital elements for healing.

Ingredients:

- 2 pounds of mixed bones (beef, chicken, or fish)
- 2 carrots, roughly chopped
- 2 celery stalks, roughly chopped

- 1 onion, quartered
- 2 tbsp apple cider vinegar
- Herbs (optional)
- Water

Preparation:

1. Place bones in a large pot and cover with water. Add apple cidervinegar.
2. Bring to a boil, then reduce to a simmer. Skim off any scum thatforms on the surface.
3. Add vegetables and optional herbs.
4. Simmer for 12-24 hours, adding water as needed to keep bonescovered.
5. Strain the broth and store in the refrigerator or freezer.

How to Use: Warm bone broth, one to two cups a day, can help boost immunity and speed the healing process from cold and flu symptoms.

Honey-Thyme Cough Syrup

Intended Use: The natural expectorant qualities of thyme combined with the soothing smoothness of honey helps to ease coughing and soothe sore throats.

Ingredients:

- ¼ cup dried thyme
- 1 cup water
- 1 cup honey

Preparation:

1. Boil water and pour over dried thyme. Let steep for 20 minutes.
2. Strain the thyme leaves and pour the thyme-infused water into asaucepan.
3. Add honey and heat over low heat until well combined, stirringfrequently.
4. Pour the syrup into a clean jar and let it cool before sealing.

How to Use: Take 1 tsp of syrup as needed to relieve coughing andsoothe sore throats. Store in the refrigerator for up to a month.

capsules of oregano oil

Intended Use: Strong antibacterial qualities of oregano oil can aid in the defense against cold and flu viruses.

Ingredients:

- Oregano essential oil
- Olive oil or coconut oil
- Empty capsules

Preparation:

1. Dilute oregano essential oil with olive oil or coconut oil at a ratio of1:3.
2. Using a dropper, carefully fill empty capsules with the oil mixture.
3. Seal the capsules.

How to Use: When you first notice any signs of a cold or flu, take one capsule twice a day with meals. Keep going for up to five days. Note: Before using, especially if you're pregnant, breastfeeding, or on other drugs, speak with a healthcare professional.

Honey-Garlic Immune-Supporting Paste

Intended Use: strengthens the immune system with the antiviral qualities of garlic and the calming effects of honey.

Ingredients:

- 3-4 cloves of garlic, finely minced or crushed
- 2 tbsp honey

Preparation:

1. Combine minced garlic and honey in a small bowl.
2. Mix thoroughly until you get a consistent paste.
3. Let the mixture sit for a few hours or overnight to enhance itspotency.

How to Use: When symptoms of the flu or cold appear, take a ½ tsp of the paste two to three times a day. Never take anything on an empty stomach.

Citrus Salad Packed with Vitamin C

Intended Use: A light salad that is rich in vitamin C from citrus fruits, which boosts immunity and lessens the intensity of cold and flu symptoms.

Ingredients:

- 2 oranges, peeled and sliced
- 1 grapefruit, peeled and sliced
- 1 tbsp chopped mint leaves
- Drizzle of honey (optional)

Preparation:

1. Arrange orange and grapefruit slices on a plate.
2. Sprinkle with chopped mint leaves.
3. Drizzle with honey if desired for added sweetness.

How to Use: During the cold and flu season, include this citrus salad in your regular meals to increase your consumption of vitamin C.

HEALTH DIGESTIVE

Digestive Tea with Peppermint and Fennel

Intended Use: The carminative qualities of fennel and the antispasmodic qualities of peppermint help to ease stomach pain and facilitate digestion.

Ingredients:

- 1 tsp dried fennel seeds
- 1 tsp dried peppermint leaves
- 1 cup boiling water

Preparation:

1. Place fennel seeds and peppermint leaves in a tea infuser or directlyin a cup.
2. Pour boiling water over the herbs and cover.
3. Steep for 10 minutes, then strain.
4. Drink warm.

How to Use: Drink a cup of this tea to help with digestion after meals or whenever you feel uncomfortable in your stomach.

Probiotic Bowl of Yogurt

Intended Use: Enhances gut flora with live probiotics found in yogurt,supporting overall digestive health.

Ingredients:

- 1 cup organic plain yogurt (ensure it contains live cultures)
- ½ cup fresh berries
- 1 tbsp ground flaxseed
- 1 tbsp honey (optional)

Preparation:

1. Spoon yogurt into a bowl.
2. Top with fresh berries and sprinkle with ground flaxseed.
3. Drizzle with honey for added sweetness if desired.

How to Use: Include in your regular breakfast regimen to promote digestion and intestinal health.

Digestive Bone Broth

Intended Use: has a high collagen content that helps mend the digestive system and promote gut health by repairing the intestinal lining.

Ingredients:

- 2 pounds of mixed bones (chicken, beef, or fish)
- 2 carrots, chopped
- 2 celery stalks, chopped
- 1 onion, chopped
- 2 tbsp apple cider vinegar
- Herbs such as thyme and rosemary
- Water to cover

Preparation:

1. Place bones in a large pot and cover with water. Add apple cidervinegar to help leach minerals from the bones.
2. Add chopped vegetables and herbs.
3. Bring to a boil, then reduce heat and simmer for 12-24 hours. Skimoff any foam or impurities that rise to the top.
4. Strain the broth through a fine mesh sieve and store in therefrigerator or freezer.

How to Use: To maintain digestive health, drink one cup of bone broth every day, either on its own or as a foundation for soups and stews.

Hot Lemon Water

Intended Use: helps remove toxins from the digestive tract and stimulates the enzymes involved in digestion.

Ingredients:

- Juice of ½ lemon
- 1 cup warm water

Preparation:

1. Squeeze the juice of half a lemon into a cup of warm water.
2. Stir to mix and drink warm.

How to Use: On an empty stomach, have your morning beverage to help your digestive system get going.

Vinegar and Apple Cider Salad Dressing

Intended Use: Because of apple cider vinegar's acidic and probiotic qualities, it enhances digestion and raises stomach acid.

Ingredients:

- ¼ cup apple cider vinegar (with "the mother")
- ¾ cup extra virgin olive oil
- 1 tsp mustard
- 1 tsp honey
- Salt and pepper to taste

Preparation:

1. In a jar, combine apple cider vinegar, olive oil, mustard, and honey.
2. Seal the jar and shake vigorously until well combined.
3. Season with salt and pepper to taste.

How to Use: Use this combination to dress salads and add digestive assistance to everyday meals.

Calming Aloe Vera Tea

Intended Use: Aloe vera's anti-inflammatory qualities soothe the digestive system and promote healing.

Ingredients:

- 2 tbsp of edible aloe vera gel
- 1 cup water or coconut water
- Juice of ½ lime

Preparation:

1. Blend aloe vera gel with water or coconut water until smooth.
2. Add lime juice and blend again.

3. Serve chilled for a refreshing digestive aid.

How to Use: Drink once daily, preferably in the morning, to supportdigestive health and soothe irritation.

Ginger Zinger Supplement

Intended Use: Strengthens digestion and eases nausea because to ginger's strong anti-inflammatory qualities.

Ingredients:

- 1 inch fresh ginger root
- Juice of 1 lemon
- ½ tsp cayenne pepper
- 1 tsp honey (optional)
- ¼ cup water

Preparation:

1. Blend ginger root with water until smooth.
2. Strain the mixture to extract ginger juice.
3. Mix ginger juice with lemon juice, cayenne pepper, and honey ifusing.
4. Drink immediately.

How to Use: Consume this shot in the morning or before meals to enhance digestive function.

Smoothie with Kefir

Intended Use: offers an abundance of probiotics to help maintain a healthy gut flora and digestive system.

Ingredients:

- 1 cup kefir
- ½ banana
- ½ cup mixed berries
- 1 tbsp chia seeds

Preparation:

1. Combine kefir, banana, berries, and chia seeds in a blender.
2. Blend until smooth.
3. Serve immediately for best taste and nutritional value.

How to Use: To enhance your probiotic consumption, have this smoothie for morning or as a snack.

Dandelion Root Bitters for Digesting

Intended Use: Enhances digestion by stimulating the formation of bile and supporting liver function with dandelion root.

Ingredients:

- 2 tbsp dried dandelion root
- 1 cup vodka or apple cider vinegar (for a non-alcoholic version)
- 1 tsp orange peel
- 1 tsp ginger root

Preparation:

1. Combine dandelion root, orange peel, and ginger root in a jar.
2. Cover with vodka or apple cider vinegar.
3. Seal the jar and let it sit in a cool, dark place for 2-4 weeks, shakingoccasionally.
4. Strain the mixture and store in a clean bottle.

How to Use: To aid with digestion, take one or two tbsp before meals.

Rich in Prebiotic Fiber Oatmeal

Intended Use: Supports gut health with a high-fiber meal that feedsbeneficial gut bacteria, enhancing digestive health.

Ingredients:

- 1 cup rolled oats
- 2 cups water or almond milk
- 1 tbsp ground flaxseeds
- ½ apple, diced
- Cinnamon to taste

Preparation:

1. Cook oats in water or almond milk according to package instructions.
2. Stir in ground flaxseeds and diced apple during the last few minutesof cooking.
3. Sprinkle with cinnamon before serving.

How to Use: For everyday digestive health support and to keep a balanced and healthy gut flora, have this high-fiber oatmeal for breakfast.

COMPOUNDNESS GASTROINTESTINAL

Ginger and Peppermint Digestive Tea

Intended Use: relieves stomach pain, lessens bloating, and eases digestive discomfort.

Ingredients:

- 1 tsp dried peppermint leaves
- 1 tsp grated fresh ginger
- 1 cup boiling water

Preparation:

1. Place peppermint leaves and grated ginger in a tea infuser or directlyinto a cup.
2. Pour boiling water over the leaves and ginger.
3. Cover and let steep for 10 minutes.
4. Strain (if needed) and serve warm.

How to Use: Especially after meals, drink this tea two to three times a day to help with digestion and ease pain.

Fennel Seed Aid for Digestion

Intended Use: relieves the cramping, bloating, and gas related to digestive problems.

Ingredients:

- 1 tsp fennel seeds
- 1 cup boiling water

Preparation:

1. Crush the fennel seeds slightly to release their oil.
2. Place the crushed seeds in a cup and pour boiling water over them.
3. Cover and let steep for 10 minutes.
4. Strain and drink warm.

How to Use: After meals, sip on a cup of fennel seed tea to aid with digestion and avoid pain.

Bone Broth for Healing the Gut

Intended Use: Collagen, amino acids, and minerals are used to nourish the digestive system and promote gut healing.

Ingredients:

- 2 pounds mixed beef bones (marrow and knuckle bones)
- 2 carrots, chopped
- 2 celery stalks, chopped
- 1 onion, quartered
- 2 tbsp apple cider vinegar
- Water to cover
- Salt to taste

Preparation:

1. Place bones in a large pot and cover with cold water. Add apple cidervinegar; let sit for 30 minutes.
2. Add vegetables to the pot. Bring to a boil, then reduce to a simmer.
3. Simmer for 12-24 hours, skimming foam and impurities from thesurface.
4. Strain the broth, season with salt, and cool.
5. Store in the refrigerator for up to 5 days or freeze for longer storage.

How to Use: Drink one cup of warm bone broth every day to promote comfort and good digestion.

Aloe Vera and Honey Rejuvenating Cocktail

Intended Use: helps heal the lining of the gastrointestinal tract and calms troubled stomachs.

Ingredients:

- 2 tbsp of pure aloe vera gel (ensure it's edible)
- 1 tbsp honey
- 1 cup water

Preparation:

1. Mix aloe vera gel and honey in a glass of water until fully dissolved.
2. Stir well to ensure a uniform mixture.

How to Use: Consume once daily on an empty stomach for gastrointestinalcomfort and health.

Comfort Herbal Digestive Capsules

Intended Use: offers a combination of herbs that are well-known for promoting digestive health and relieving pain.

Ingredients:

- Dried peppermint leaf powder
- Dried ginger root powder
- Dried fennel seed powder
- Empty capsules

Preparation:

1. In a bowl, mix equal parts of peppermint, ginger, and fennelpowders.
2. Fill empty capsules with the herbal mixture using a capsule filler or asmall spoon.
3. Store the filled capsules in a cool, dry place.

How to Use: Take one or two capsules as needed to relieve upset stomach; do not take more than six capsules in a day.

Hot Water with Lemon and Cinnamon

Intended Use: increases gastrointestinal motility and stimulates digestion enzymes.

Ingredients:

- Juice of ½ lemon
- ½ tsp cinnamon
- 1 cup warm water

Preparation:

1. Add lemon juice and cinnamon to warm water.
2. Stir well to combine.

How to Use: Take one or two capsules as needed to relieve upset stomach; do not take more than six capsules in a day.

Digestive Smoothie with Papaya

Intended Use: includes papain, a papaya enzyme that aids in protein digestion, minimizing bloating and enhancing digestive health.

Ingredients:

- 1 cup fresh papaya, chopped
- ½ banana
- 1 cup coconut water
- 1 tbsp lime juice
- A handful of ice

Preparation:

1. Place papaya, banana, coconut water, lime juice, and ice in a blender.
2. Blend until smooth.
3. Serve immediately.

How to Use: Have this smoothie in the morning or right before meals to help with digestion and to soothe your stomach.

Rich in Probiotics Sauerkraut

Intended Use: Enhances gut flora balance and supports overall digestivehealth with natural probiotics.

Ingredients:

- 1 medium head cabbage, shredded
- 1 tbsp sea salt

Preparation:

1. Mix cabbage and salt in a large bowl. Massage until cabbage releasesits juice.
2. Pack cabbage tightly into a clean mason jar, pressing down untiljuices cover the cabbage.
3. Cover the jar with a cloth and secure with a rubber band.
4. Let the jar sit at room temperature for 3-10 days. Check daily,pressing down the cabbage if it rises above its liquid.
5. Once fermented, seal the jar and store in the refrigerator.

How to Use: Include a small portion of sauerkraut in your daily diet tomaintain healthy digestion and gut flora.

Berry-Kefir Digestive Parfait

Intended Use: combines berries' fiber and kefir's probiotics to create a delicious treat that improves digestive health.

Ingredients:

- 1 cup plain kefir
- ½ cup mixed berries (blueberries, strawberries, raspberries)
- 1 tbsp chia seeds
- Honey (optional, for sweetness)

Preparation:

1. In a glass, layer kefir, berries, and chia seeds.
2. Repeat the layers until all ingredients are used.
3. Drizzle with honey if desired.

How to Use: Savor it for breakfast or as a snack to help maintain healthy digestive tract function by combining fiber and probiotics.

Cucumber Mint Juice for Hydration

Intended Use: hydrates the body and aids with digestive health with a cool cucumber-mint combination.

Ingredients:

- 1 large cucumber, peeled and chopped
- 10 mint leaves
- Juice of 1 lime
- 1 cup water

Preparation:

1. Blend cucumber, mint leaves, lime juice, and water until smooth.
2. Strain the juice for a smoother texture, if desired.
3. Serve chilled.

How to Use: Drink this juice throughout the day to stay hydrated and supportyour digestive system, particularly in hot weather or after workouts.

RELIEF FROM HEADACHE AND MIGRAINE

Ginger Tea for Instant Headache Relief

Intended Use: Ginger helps to relieve headaches and migraines by lowering inflammation and enhancing blood flow.

Ingredients:

- 1 inch fresh ginger root, thinly sliced
- 2 cups water
- Honey to taste

Preparation:

1. Boil water in a saucepan and add sliced ginger.
2. Simmer for 10-15 minutes.
3. Strain the tea into a cup and add honey to taste.

How to Use: Drink ginger tea at the first sign of a headache or migraine forrelief. Limit to 2-3 cups per day.

Rich in Magnesium Banana Smoothie

Intended Use: provide a sufficient supply of magnesium, which helps avoid headaches and migraines.

Ingredients:

- 1 ripe banana
- 1 cup spinach
- 1 tbsp chia seeds
- 1 cup almond milk
- A handful of almonds

Preparation:

1. Blend all ingredients together until smooth.
2. Serve immediately.

How to Use: To increase magnesium intake, drink this smoothie frequently, especially when you're experiencing headaches or migraines frequently.

Lavender and Peppermint Essential Oil for Pain Relief

Intended Use: Thanks to the calming and anti-inflammatory qualities of peppermint and lavender, it relieves headaches and migraines.

Ingredients:

- 2 tbsp almond oil (or any carrier oil like coconut or jojoba oil)
- 4 drops peppermint essential oil
- 4 drops lavender essential oil

Preparation:

1. In a small bottle, mix the almond oil with peppermint and lavender essential oils.
2. Shake well to combine.

How to Use: When a headache or migraine starts, massage a tiny bit of the oil over your forehead, temples, and back of your neck. Reapply if necessary. Steer clear of the eyes.

Feverfew Infusion to Prevent Headaches

Intended Use: uses feverfew's preventative qualities to delay the development of migraines.

Ingredients:

- 1 tsp dried feverfew leaves
- 1 cup boiling water

Preparation:

1. Place feverfew leaves in a cup and cover with boiling water.
2. Steep for 10-15 minutes, then strain.
3. Drink the infusion once cooled.

How to Use: Drink once a day to lessen your risk of migraines. Note: Women who are expecting or breastfeeding should not use feverfew.

Anti-Inflammatory Turmeric Milk

Intended Use: lessens the inflammation linked to migraines and headaches.

Ingredients:

- 1 cup almond milk
- 1 tsp turmeric powder
- ¼ tsp black pepper (to enhance absorption)
- Honey to taste

Preparation:

1. Heat almond milk in a saucepan over low heat.
2. Stir in turmeric and black pepper.
3. Remove from heat and sweeten with honey.
4. Serve warm.

How to Use: Drink in the evening before going to bed to help ease headaches and decrease inflammation.

Blend for Inhaling Essential Oils

Intended Use: reduces headache discomfort by using essential oils' aromatherapeutic properties.

Ingredients:

- 2 drops eucalyptus essential oil
- 2 drops rosemary essential oil
- 2 drops peppermint essential oil

Preparation:

1. Boil a pot of water and remove from heat.
2. Add essential oils to the hot water.
3. Lean over the pot, cover your head and the pot with a towel, andinhale the steam for 5-10 minutes.

How to Use: Use this inhalation method at the first sign of a headache forimmediate relief.

Enhance Hydration with Cucumber Water

Intended Use: increases hydration to prevent headaches caused by dehydration.

Ingredients:

- 1 cucumber, thinly sliced
- 2 liters water
- Mint leaves (optional)

Preparation:

1. Add cucumber slices (and mint if using) to a large pitcher of water.
2. Refrigerate for at least an hour to infuse.
3. Drink throughout the day.

How to Use: Make sure you drink enough, especially in the summer or after working out, to avoid headaches from dehydration.

Cayenne Pepper Pain Relief Balm

Intended Use: uses the capsaicin in cayenne pepper, which has pain-relieving qualities, to lessen headache and migraine suffering.

Ingredients:

- ¼ cup coconut oil
- 1 tsp cayenne pepper powder
- 1 tbsp beeswax pellets

Preparation:

1. Gently heat coconut oil and beeswax in a double boiler until melted.
2. Stir in cayenne pepper powder.
3. Pour mixture into a small container and let solidify.
4. Once cooled, apply a small amount to the temples and back of theneck. Avoid eye area and any open skin.

How to Use: Apply judiciously as soon as headache symptoms appear. After applying, carefully wash your hands.

Calm Lavender-Spun Lemonade

Intended Use: Lavender relaxes and calms the nervous system, which lessens the incidence of headaches and migraines.

Ingredients:

- 4 cups water

- Juice of 1 lemon
- 1 tbsp dried lavender flowers
- Honey to taste

Preparation:

1. Boil water and pour over lavender flowers to steep for about 15minutes.
2. Strain the lavender and mix the infused water with lemon juice.
3. Sweeten with honey to taste and chill in the refrigerator.
4. Serve cold.

How to Use: Have one or two cups every day to help prevent and manage headaches, particularly stress-related headaches.

Walnut and Flaxseed Pudding Packed with Omega-3

Intended Use: supplies omega-3 fatty acids from walnuts and flaxseeds, which support brain function and prevent inflammation that might cause headaches.

Ingredients:

- 2 tbsp ground flaxseeds
- ¼ cup walnuts, chopped
- 1 cup almond milk
- 1 tbsp chia seeds
- 1 banana, mashed
- Honey or maple syrup to taste

Preparation:

1. Mix almond milk, chia seeds, flaxseeds, and mashed banana in abowl.
2. Let sit for an hour or overnight in the refrigerator until it reaches apudding-like consistency.
3. Top with chopped walnuts and sweeten with honey or maple syrup asdesired.

How to Use: To avoid headaches, include anti-inflammatory omega-3 fatty acids in your diet by having this pudding for breakfast or as a snack.

HEART AND CIRCULATION

Flaxseed and Berries with Oatmeal

Intended Use: lowers cholesterol and supplies a lot of omega-3 fatty acids and antioxidants, all of which are beneficial to heart health.

Ingredients:

- 1 cup rolled oats
- 2 cups water or almond milk
- ½ cup mixed berries (blueberries, strawberries, raspberries)
- 2 tbsp ground flaxseed
- Honey or maple syrup to taste

Preparation:

1. Cook oats in water or almond milk according to package instructions.
2. Once cooked, stir in ground flaxseed.
3. Top with mixed berries and sweeten with honey or maple syrup asdesired.
4. Serve warm.

How to Use: Savor this heart-healthy oatmeal for breakfast to get your day started.

Avocado and Walnut Salad

Intended Use: provide a good dose of omega-3 fatty acids and heart-healthy monounsaturated fats.

Ingredients:

- 2 cups mixed salad greens
- 1 ripe avocado, sliced
- ½ cup walnuts, roughly chopped
- ¼ cup cherry tomatoes, halved
- Dressing: Olive oil, lemon juice, salt, and pepper

Preparation:

1. In a large salad bowl, toss together the salad greens, avocado slices,walnuts, and cherry tomatoes.

2. In a small bowl, whisk together olive oil, lemon juice, salt, andpepper to make the dressing.
3. Drizzle the dressing over the salad and toss gently to combine.

How to Use: Serve this salad as an appetizer or as a side to increase your intake of heart-healthy fats.

Sardine and Whole Grain Toast

Intended Use: provide a good dose of omega-3 fatty acids and heart-healthy monounsaturated fats.

Ingredients:

- 2 slices of whole grain bread, toasted
- 1 can of sardines in olive oil, drained
- 1 tbsp lemon juice
- Fresh herbs (parsley, dill, or chives), chopped
- Salt and pepper to taste

Preparation:

1. Mash the sardines with a fork and mix with lemon juice, choppedherbs, salt, and pepper.
2. Spread the sardine mixture evenly over the toasted whole grainbread.
3. Serve immediately.

How to Use: Savor this nutrient-dense toast for breakfast or lunch to help heart health with whole grains and important fatty acids.

Blend of Hibiscus and Green Tea

Intended Use: uses antioxidants from hibiscus and green tea, which are proven to decrease blood pressure, to improve cardiovascular health.

Ingredients:

- 1 tsp green tea leaves
- 1 tsp dried hibiscus flowers
- 1 cup boiling water
- Honey to taste (optional)

Preparation:

1. Combine green tea leaves and dried hibiscus flowers in a tea infuseror teapot.
2. Pour boiling water over the tea blend and let steep for 5 minutes.
3. Remove the infuser or strain the tea. Sweeten with honey if desired.
4. Serve hot or chilled.

How to Use: To promote heart health and decrease blood pressure, have one to two cups each day.

Heart-Sănătizing Beet Juice

Intended Use: uses beet nitrates, which lower blood pressure and enhance blood flow.

Ingredients:

- 2 medium beets, peeled and chopped
- 1 apple, cored and sliced
- ½ inch ginger, peeled
- ½ lemon, peeled
- Water (optional, for adjusting consistency)

Preparation:

1. Place all ingredients in a juicer.
2. Process until smooth. Add water if you prefer a thinner consistency.
3. Serve the juice immediately for maximum nutrient retention.

How to Use: Drink a small glass (about 8 ounces) of beet juice daily tosupport cardiovascular health.

Seed and Almond Trail Mix

Intended Use: Eat a snack high in fiber, protein, and heart-healthy fats to promote general cardiovascular wellbeing.

Ingredients:

- ½ cup almonds
- ½ cup walnuts
- ¼ cup pumpkin seeds
- ¼ cup sunflower seeds

- ¼ cup dried cranberries
- A pinch of sea salt

Preparation:

1. Combine all ingredients in a large mixing bowl.
2. Toss with a pinch of sea salt.
3. Store the trail mix in an airtight container.

How to Use: Eat this mixture as snacks to maintain your energy levels and heart health.

Pudding with Chia Seeds and Berries

Intended Use: provides a heart-healthy, high-fiber snack or dessert that is rich in omega-3 fatty acids.

Ingredients:

- ¼ cup chia seeds
- 1 cup almond milk
- 1 tbsp maple syrup or honey
- ½ tsp vanilla extract
- ½ cup mixed berries

Preparation:

1. In a bowl, whisk together chia seeds, almond milk, maple syrup orhoney, and vanilla extract until well combined.
2. Refrigerate for at least 4 hours or overnight, until it reaches a pudding-like consistency.
3. Top with mixed berries before serving.

How to Use: To benefit from this pudding's heart-healthy properties, eat it as a filling breakfast or snack.

Kale and Lentil Soup

Intended Use: offers a plentiful supply of iron, fiber, and plant-based protein for heart health.

Ingredients:

- 1 cup dried lentils, rinsed

- 4 cups vegetable broth
- 1 onion, diced
- 2 carrots, diced
- 2 stalks celery, diced
- 2 cups kale, chopped
- 2 garlic cloves, minced
- 1 tsp turmeric
- Salt and pepper to taste
- 2 tbsp olive oil

Preparation:

1. Heat olive oil in a large pot over medium heat. Add onion, carrots,and celery; cook until softened.
2. Add garlic and turmeric; cook for another minute.
3. Pour in the vegetable broth and add lentils. Bring to a boil, thenreduce heat and simmer until lentils are tender.
4. Stir in kale and cook until wilted.
5. Season with salt and pepper to taste.

How to Use: Savor this filling soup for lunch or dinner and reap the benefits of its heart-healthy components.

Dressing with Garlic and Olive Oil

Intended Use: benefits heart health by decreasing cholesterol and acting as an anti-inflammatory when combined with olive oil.

Ingredients:

- ½ cup extra virgin olive oil
- 2 cloves garlic, minced
- 2 tbsp apple cider vinegar
- 1 tsp mustard
- Salt and pepper to taste

Preparation:

1. In a small bowl, whisk together olive oil, minced garlic, apple cidervinegar, and mustard.

2. Season with salt and pepper to taste.
3. Store in an airtight container in the refrigerator.

How to Use: To add additional heart-healthy fats and garlic to your diet, use this dressing as a marinade or on salads.

Heart-Healthy Quinoa and Spinach Salad

Intended Use: rich in vitamins, minerals, and antioxidants to promote heart health and lower inflammation.

Ingredients:

- 1 cup cooked quinoa
- 2 cups spinach, chopped
- ¼ cup sliced almonds
- ¼ cup feta cheese, crumbled
- ¼ cup pomegranate seeds
- Dressing: Lemon juice, olive oil, salt, and pepper

Preparation:

1. In a large salad bowl, combine cooked quinoa, chopped spinach, sliced almonds, crumbled feta cheese, and pomegranate seeds.
2. In a small bowl, whisk together lemon juice, olive oil, salt, andpepper to create the dressing.
3. Drizzle the dressing over the salad and toss gently to combine.

How to Use: For a nutrient-dense, heart-healthy lunch or supper, serve this salad as the main course.

HYPERTENSIVE BALANCE

Chasteberry Tea

Intended Use: Because chasteberry (Vitex) affects hormone levels, it helps regulate menstrual cycles and relieves PMS and menopausal symptoms.

Ingredients:

- 1 tsp dried chasteberry
- 1 cup boiling water

Preparation:

1. Place dried chasteberry in a tea infuser or directly in a cup.
2. Pour boiling water over the chasteberry.
3. Cover and steep for 10 minutes.
4. Strain the tea into another cup if you've not used an infuser.
5. Drink warm.

How to Use: To promote hormonal balance, drink one cup of chasteberry tea every day, especially in the second half of the menstrual cycle.

Berry and Flaxseed Breakfast Bowl

Intended Use: supplies antioxidants from berries and phytoestrogens from flaxseeds to assist hormone health and cleansing.

Ingredients:

- ¼ cup ground flaxseeds
- 1 cup Greek yogurt or plant-based yogurt
- ½ cup fresh berries (blueberries, strawberries, raspberries)
- 1 tbsp honey or maple syrup
- A sprinkle of hemp seeds (optional)

Preparation:

1. In a bowl, mix the Greek yogurt with ground flaxseeds.
2. Top with fresh berries and a drizzle of honey or maple syrup.
3. Add a sprinkle of hemp seeds for extra nutrition (optional).

4. Mix gently before eating.

How to Use: Eat this breakfast dish to start your day off right with a meal that balances your hormones.

Smoothie with Maca Root

Intended Use: Maca root, well-known for its adaptogenic qualities, supports hormonal balance and increases vitality.

Ingredients:

- 1 tbsp maca powder
- 1 banana
- 1 cup almond milk
- 1 tbsp almond butter
- ½ tsp cinnamon
- Ice cubes (optional)

Preparation:

1. Place maca powder, banana, almond milk, almond butter, andcinnamon in a blender.
2. Add ice cubes for a chilled smoothie (optional).
3. Blend until smooth and creamy.
4. Serve immediately for best taste and nutrient retention.

How to Use: Drink this smoothie in the morning or early afternoon to help maintain energy levels and hormonal balance all day.

Herbal Supplemental Ashwagandha

Intended Use: Enhances adrenal health and lowers stress with ashwagandha, an adaptogen that aids in cortisol regulation.

Ingredients:

- Ashwagandha powder
- Empty capsules

Preparation:

1. Invest in premium, organic ashwagandha powder from a reliable supplier.

2. Fill empty capsules with ashwagandha powder using a capsule machine or manually with a small spoon.
3. Store the filled capsules in a cool, dry place.

How to Use: Take one or two ashwagandha capsules per day, ideally with meals and drinks, to help with hormone balance and stress management.

Salad with Avocado and Seeds

Intended Use: supplies fiber and good fats from seeds and avocados to aid in the production and regulation of hormones.

Ingredients:

- 1 ripe avocado, sliced
- 2 cups mixed salad greens
- ¼ cup mixed seeds (pumpkin, sunflower, sesame)
- Dressing: 2 tbsp extra virgin olive oil, 1 tbsp lemon juice,salt, and pepper

Preparation:

1. In a large salad bowl, toss together the salad greens and slicedavocado.
2. Sprinkle mixed seeds over the salad.
3. In a small bowl, whisk together olive oil, lemon juice, salt, andpepper to create the dressing.
4. Drizzle the dressing over the salad before serving.

How to Use: With nutrient-dense ingredients, enjoy this salad as a satisfying lunch to maintain hormonal balance.

Smoothie with Spirulina Energy Boost

Intended Use: Contains a high-nutrient superfood that supports thyroid function and general energy levels: spirulina.

Ingredients:

- 1 tsp spirulina powder
- 1 banana
- 1 cup spinach
- 1 tbsp almond butter

- 1 cup almond milk
- Ice cubes (optional)

Preparation:

1. Place all ingredients in a blender, adding ice cubes if a coldersmoothie is preferred.
2. Blend until smooth.
3. Serve immediately for maximum freshness and nutrient content.

How to Use: To improve thyroid function and to increase energy and support hormonal health in general, drink this smoothie in the morning or before working out.

Green Leafy Vegetable Stir-Fry

Intended Use: cruciferous vegetables improve the metabolism of estrogen and support hormonal balance.

Ingredients:

- 2 cups mixed green leafy and cruciferous vegetables (kale, broccoli,Brussels sprouts)
- 1 tbsp olive oil
- 2 cloves garlic, minced
- Salt and pepper to taste
- Lemon juice (optional)

Preparation:

1. Heat olive oil in a pan over medium heat.
2. Add minced garlic and sauté for 1 minute until fragrant.
3. Add the mixed vegetables to the pan, stir-frying until tender but stillvibrant.
4. Season with salt and pepper. Finish with a squeeze of lemon juice forextra flavor.
5. Serve warm.

How to Use: Add this stir-fry to your meals two or three times a week to help with hormonal balance and detoxification.

Seaweed Salad for Healthy Thyroid Function

Intended Use: seaweed's natural iodine, which is essential for the creation of hormones, supports thyroid function.

Ingredients:

- 1 cup dried seaweed (wakame or arame), rehydrated
- 1 cucumber, thinly sliced
- 2 tbsp rice vinegar
- 1 tbsp soy sauce
- 1 tsp sesame oil
- Sesame seeds for garnish

Preparation:

1. Rehydrate dried seaweed according to package instructions, thendrain.
2. In a bowl, mix rehydrated seaweed and sliced cucumber.
3. In a separate bowl, whisk together rice vinegar, soy sauce, andsesame oil for the dressing.
4. Pour dressing over seaweed and cucumber, tossing to coat.
5. Garnish with sesame seeds before serving.

How to Use: Eat this salad regularly, 2-3 times a week, to provide the bodywith essential nutrients for thyroid and hormonal health.

Lemon Balm Herbal Tea

Intended Use: Lemon balm helps to maintain a tranquil mood and lower anxiety; it is also good for hormone balance.

Ingredients:

- 1 tbsp dried lemon balm leaves
- 1 cup boiling water

Preparation:

1. Place lemon balm leaves in a tea infuser or directly in a mug.
2. Pour boiling water over the leaves and let steep for 5-10 minutes.
3. Remove the infuser or strain the tea.
4. Drink warm or allow to cool for a refreshing beverage.

How to Use: Drink 1-2 cups of lemon balm tea every day to help with hormone balance and relaxation.

Pomegranate Juice for Equilibrium Hormones

Intended Use: uses pomegranate's natural ingredients to balance estrogen levels, which is good for both men and women.

Ingredients:

- 2 pomegranates
- 1 cup water (optional, to adjust taste)

Preparation:

1. Cut the pomegranates and remove the seeds.
2. Blend the seeds with a cup of water if a less concentrated juice isdesired.
3. Strain the mixture to remove the pulp and seeds.
4. Serve the juice chilled or at room temperature.

How to Use: Every day, have a small glass of pomegranate juice to help with hormone balance and to get the advantages of antioxidants.

BRONCHIAL AND LUNG HEALTH

Mullein Tea to Assist with Respiration

Intended Use: With mullein's expectorant qualities, it soothes the respiratory system and promotes lung health.

Ingredients:

- 1-2 tsps dried mullein leaves
- 1 cup boiling water
- Honey (optional)

Preparation:

1. Place mullein leaves in a tea infuser or directly in a mug.
2. Pour boiling water over the leaves and cover the mug.
3. Steep for 10-15 minutes.
4. Strain the tea into another cup if leaves were added directly.
5. Add honey to taste, if desired.

How to Use: To improve lung health and ease respiratory problems, have two to three cups each day.

Inhaling Eucalyptus Steam

Intended Use: opens airways and makes breathing easier because to eucalyptus's decongestant qualities.

Ingredients:

- 3-5 drops eucalyptus essential oil
- A bowl of boiling water

Preparation:

1. Add eucalyptus essential oil to a bowl of boiling water.
2. Lean over the bowl and cover your head and the bowl with a towel totrap the steam.
3. Inhale deeply for 5-10 minutes.

How to Use: Once or twice a day, as required, use a steam inhalation to help promote lung health and reduce congestion.

Root Licorice Lung Tonic

Intended Use: Licorice root calms inflamed bronchial passageways and supports lung health.

Ingredients:

- 1 tsp dried licorice root
- 1 cup boiling water

Preparation:

1. Place licorice root in a cup and cover with boiling water.
2. Steep for 10 minutes.
3. Strain and drink the tea warm.

How to Use: Consume 1-2 cups daily to support respiratory health. Avoid long-term use and consult with a healthcare provider if you have high blood pressure.

Honey-Thyme Cough Syrup

Intended Use: uses thyme's antibacterial qualities to soothe coughs and promote bronchial health.

Ingredients:

- ¼ cup dried thyme
- 1 cup water
- 1 cup honey

Preparation:

1. Boil water and pour over the dried thyme. Let it steep for 15 minutes.
2. Strain the thyme from the water and mix the thyme-infused waterwith honey in a saucepan.
3. Heat gently until well combined, then allow to cool.
4. Transfer to a jar and seal tightly.

How to Use: Take 1 tsp up to 4 times daily if you have bronchial discomfort or a cough.

Drink with Turmeric and Ginger for Inflammation

Intended Use: reduces respiratory system irritation by using the anti-inflammatory qualities of turmeric and ginger.

Ingredients:

- 1 inch fresh ginger, grated
- 1 tsp turmeric powder
- Juice of 1 lemon
- 1 tbsp honey
- 2 cups hot water

Preparation:

1. Add ginger, turmeric, and lemon juice to hot water.
2. Allow to steep for 10-15 minutes.
3. Strain into a cup and stir in honey.

How to Use: Warm beverages should be had one to two times a day, particularly in the winter or when you're having respiratory problems.

Pine Needle Cold Sore Relief

Intended Use: Pine needles' antibacterial qualities and vitamin C support respiratory health and ease coughing.

Ingredients:

- A handful of fresh pine needles (from a safe, edible variety)
- 2 cups water
- Honey to taste

Preparation:

1. Rinse pine needles and chop them finely.
2. Boil water and add the pine needles.
3. Simmer for 20-30 minutes.
4. Strain the liquid and add honey to taste.

How to Use: Warm one cup should be had twice a day to promote respiratory health and ease coughing.

Syrup for Onions and Honey Respiratory

Intended Use: With onion and honey, it relieves respiratory irritation and functions as a natural expectorant.

Ingredients:

- 1 medium onion, chopped finely
- ½ cup honey

Preparation:

1. Place chopped onion in a bowl and cover with honey.
2. Let the mixture sit overnight at room temperature to allow the onion to infuse into the honey.
3. The next day, strain the mixture to remove the onion pieces, retainingthe infused honey.
4. Transfer the onion-infused honey to a clean jar and seal tightly.

How to Use: Take one tsp of this syrup, up to four times daily, to help maintain respiratory health, ease sore throats, and reduce coughs. This treatment works especially well when it's cold and flu season or if you're having trouble breathing.

Peppermint Bronchial Soothing Tea

Intended Use: helps breathing by relieving bronchial inflammation and using peppermint's calming and anti-inflammatory properties.

Ingredients:

- 1 tbsp dried peppermint leaves
- 1 cup boiling water

Preparation:

1. Steep peppermint leaves in boiling water for 10 minutes.
2. Strain and serve the tea warm.

How to Use: Drink one to two glasses per day to facilitate easy breathing and relax the respiratory tract.

Alkaline Water and Sea Moss

Intended Use: Because sea moss contains a high concentration of minerals, it nourishes the body and promotes respiratory health.

Ingredients:

- 2 tbsp sea moss gel
- 1 cup alkaline water
- Juice of ½ lemon

Preparation:

1. Prepare sea moss gel according to package instructions, if not pre-made.
2. In a glass, combine the sea moss gel with alkaline water.
3. Squeeze the juice of half a lemon into the mixture and stir well.

How to Use: Drink once a day in the morning on an empty stomach to help maintain respiratory health and general well-being. Numerous minerals and vitamins found in sea moss are known to boost lung and immunological function.

Capsules of Oregano Oil for Respiratory Health

Intended Use: Supports the immune system and provides antimicrobialbenefits to the respiratory system with oregano oil.

Ingredients:

- Oregano essential oil
- Olive oil (if diluting is necessary)
- Empty capsules

Preparation:

1. If using pure oregano essential oil, dilute it with olive oil at a ratio of1:1 due to its potency.
2. Using a dropper, fill each empty capsule with the oregano oilmixture.
3. Seal the capsules.

How to Use: Take one capsule with meals twice a day. Maintain respiratory health for as long as two weeks, especially when there's a higher chance of respiratory problems. Because oregano oil is strong, it's best to start with a smaller dosage and see how well you tolerate it. Before beginning any new supplement regimen, always get medical advice, especially if you are using medication or already have health issues.

MEMORY IMPROVEMENT

Ginkgo Biloba Extract

Intended Use: Known for its capacity to promote cognitive function, ginkgo biloba supports brain health and enhances memory.

Ingredients:

- Ginkgo Biloba leaves or pre-made Ginkgo Biloba extract
- Capsule machine and empty capsules (if making your own)

Preparation:

1. If using leaves, dry and grind them into a fine powder.
2. Use a capsule machine to fill empty capsules with Ginkgo Bilobapowder.
3. If using pre-made extract, follow the dosage instructions on thepackaging.

How to Use: As advised by a healthcare professional, the product instructions, or both, take one capsule in the morning.

Blueberry and Walnut Brain Health Smoothie

Intended Use: antioxidants from blueberries and omega-3 fatty acids from walnuts nourish the brain and enhance memory.

Ingredients:

- ¼ cup walnuts
- ½ cup blueberries
- 1 banana
- 1 cup spinach leaves
- 1 cup almond milk

Preparation:

1. Combine all ingredients in a blender.
2. Blend until smooth.
3. Serve immediately.

How to Use: Savor this smoothie for breakfast or as a wholesome snack to maintain mental well-being all day.

Memory-Boosting Rosemary and Lemon Tea

Intended Use: uses the reviving clarity of lemon and the cognitively supporting qualities of rosemary to improve memory and attention.

Ingredients:

- 1 tsp dried rosemary leaves
- 1 cup boiling water
- Juice of ½ lemon
- Honey (optional)

Preparation:

1. Place rosemary leaves in a cup and cover with boiling water.
2. Steep for 5-10 minutes.
3. Strain the tea and add lemon juice.
4. Sweeten with honey if desired.

How to Use: Take this tea in the afternoon to clear your head or in the morning to get your day going.

Curcumin Supplements for Improving Memory

Intended Use: uses turmeric's anti-inflammatory and antioxidant characteristics to enhance memory and cognitive performance.

Ingredients:

- Curcumin (turmeric) powder
- Black pepper extract (to enhance absorption)
- Empty capsules

Preparation:

1. Mix curcumin powder with a small amount of black pepper extract.
2. Fill empty capsules with the mixture.
3. Seal the capsules.

How to Use: Take one capsule daily with meals to enhance memory andcognitive function.

Tea for Sage Memory Enhancement

Intended Use: uses sage's neuroprotective qualities to improve cognitive function and memory retention.

Ingredients:

- 1 tbsp dried sage leaves
- 1 cup boiling water
- Honey (optional)

Preparation:

1. Steep sage leaves in boiling water for 5-10 minutes.
2. Strain and add honey if desired.
3. Drink warm.

How to Use: Drink one cup of sage tea every day, particularly when you're doing a lot of cerebral work.

Omega-3 Rich Flaxseed Oil Dressing

Intended Use: Supports brain health and cognitive function with the omega-3 fatty acids found in flaxseed oil.

Ingredients:

- ¼ cup flaxseed oil
- Juice of 1 lemon
- 2 tsps Dijon mustard
- Salt and pepper to taste

Preparation:

1. Whisk together flaxseed oil, lemon juice, Dijon mustard, salt, and pepper.
2. Store in a sealed container in the refrigerator.

How to Use: For better memory and cognitive function, use this dressing on salads or vegetables on a daily basis to provide omega-3 fatty acids to your diet.

Memory Boosting Avocado and Chia Seed Pudding

Intended Use: provides fiber from chia seeds and healthy fats from avocado to support memory and brain health.

Ingredients:

- 1 ripe avocado
- 2 tbsp chia seeds
- 1 cup coconut milk
- 1 tbsp honey or maple syrup
- ½ tsp vanilla extract

Preparation:

1. Mash the avocado in a bowl.
2. Mix in chia seeds, coconut milk, sweetener, and vanilla extract.
3. Let the mixture sit in the refrigerator for an hour until it thickens intoa pudding.

How to Use: Savor this pudding for dessert or as a snack to help maintain cognitive and memory function.

Brahmi (Bacopa Monnieri) Herbal Tonic

Intended Use: uses sage's neuroprotective qualities to improve cognitive function and memory retention.

Ingredients:

- 1 tsp dried Brahmi leaves
- 1 cup boiling water

Preparation:

1. Steep Brahmi leaves in boiling water for 10 minutes.
2. Strain and drink warm.

How to Use: Once a day, sip this tonic to help maintain cognitive and memory function.

Almond and Pumpkin Seed Snack Mix

Intended Use: supplies zinc and good fats to promote brain health and memory enhancement.

Ingredients:

- ½ cup pumpkin seeds

- ½ cup almonds
- A pinch of sea salt

Preparation:

1. Mix pumpkin seeds and almonds together.
2. Lightly toast the mix in a dry skillet over medium heat until fragrant.
3. Sprinkle with sea salt and let cool.

How to Use: Enjoy this snack mix as a midday snack to support cognitivefunction and memory.

Enhancer of Memory Matcha Green Tea

Intended Use: enhances concentration and memory thanks to matcha green tea's antioxidants.

Ingredients:

- 1 tsp matcha green tea powder
- 1 cup hot water
- Honey or maple syrup (optional)

Preparation:

1. Sift matcha powder into a cup to remove any lumps.
2. Add a small amount of hot water and whisk until a paste forms.
3. Add the rest of the water and whisk until frothy.
4. Sweeten with honey or maple syrup if desired.

How to Use: Take a cup of matcha green tea in the morning or early afternoon to improve cognitive function, memory, and attention.

MENSTRUAL SUPPORT

Raspberry Leaf Tea to Help with Menstruation

Intended Use: The toning characteristics of raspberry leaf help to improve uterine health and alleviate period cramps.

Ingredients:

- 1 tbsp dried raspberry leaves
- 1 cup boiling water
- Honey (optional)

Preparation:

1. Place raspberry leaves in a cup or tea infuser.
2. Pour boiling water over the leaves and cover.
3. Steep for 10-15 minutes.
4. Strain and add honey to taste, if desired.

How to Use: onset drinking 1-2 cups per day a week before the onset of your period to help promote the health of your uterus and relieve menstrual cramps.

Tea with Chamomile for Relaxation

Intended Use: Because chamomile has relaxing effects, it helps to induce relaxation and ease period cramps.

Ingredients:

- 2 tsps dried chamomile flowers
- 1 cup boiling water
- Honey or lemon (optional)

Preparation:

1. Add chamomile flowers to a cup or tea infuser.
2. Pour boiling water over chamomile and cover.
3. Steep for 5-10 minutes.
4. Strain and add honey or lemon to taste, if desired.

How to Use: Sip one or two cups in the evening or if you're having menstrual pain to help relax and reduce cramps.

Rich in Magnesium Banana Smoothie

Intended Use: benefits menstrual health and lessens cramps by relaxing muscles with magnesium.

Ingredients:

- 1 ripe banana
- 1 cup spinach
- 1 tbsp almond butter
- 1 cup almond milk
- 1 tbsp chia seeds

Preparation:

1. Combine all ingredients in a blender.
2. Blend until smooth.
3. Serve immediately.

How to Use: Drink this smoothie every day to boost your intake of magnesium and lessen cramps, particularly in the second half of your menstrual cycle.

Drink of Ginger Anti-Inflammatory for Menstrual Pain

Intended Use: Ginger's inherent anti-inflammatory qualities help to reduce inflammation and menstruation discomfort.

Ingredients:

- 1 inch fresh ginger, grated
- 2 cups water
- Juice of half a lemon
- 1 tsp honey

Preparation:

1. Boil water and add grated ginger.
2. Simmer for 10 minutes.
3. Strain the mixture and add lemon juice and honey.

4. Stir well and drink warm.

How to Use: Take as required to relieve menstrual discomfort; during your period, take up to three times a day.

Tea with Fennel Seeds for Bloating

Intended Use: Alleviates bloating and digestive discomfort associated withmenstruation using fennel seeds.

Ingredients:

- 1 tsp fennel seeds
- 1 cup boiling water

Preparation:

1. Crush the fennel seeds slightly to release their oil.
2. Place in a cup and cover with boiling water.
3. Steep for 10 minutes.
4. Strain and drink warm.

How to Use: During your menstrual cycle, drink one to two cups every day to help with bloating and upset stomach.

Blended Peppermint Oil for Abdominal Massage

Intended Use: Menstrual cramps and stomach pain can be relieved by peppermint oil's calming effects.

Ingredients:

- 2 tbsp carrier oil (such as coconut or almond oil)
- 4-5 drops peppermint essential oil

Preparation:

1. Mix peppermint essential oil with the carrier oil thoroughly.
2. Store in a glass bottle.

How to Use: When you have period cramps, gently massage in circular strokes across your belly. Use sparingly and keep out of delicate regions.

Maca Powder for Enhanced Energy

Intended Use: Maca powder helps maintain energy levels and hormonal balance during menstruation.

Ingredients:

- 1 tsp maca powder
- 1 cup your favorite smoothie or juice

Preparation:

1. Add maca powder to your smoothie or juice.
2. Blend well to ensure the maca is fully mixed.

How to Use: Take one capsule daily, preferably first thing in the morning, to help maintain hormonal balance and energy levels during your menstrual cycle.

Iron-Packed Lentil and Spinach Soup

Intended Use: nutrient-rich soup that promotes blood health and restores iron lost during menstruation.

Ingredients:

- 1 cup lentils
- 2 cups spinach, chopped
- 1 onion, diced
- 2 cloves garlic, minced
- 4 cups vegetable broth
- 1 tbsp olive oil
- Salt and pepper to taste

Preparation:

1. Heat olive oil in a pot over medium heat. Add onion and garlic,cooking until soft.
2. Add lentils and vegetable broth. Bring to a boil, then simmer untillentils are tender.
3. Stir in spinach and cook until wilted.
4. Season with salt and pepper.
5. Blend partially or fully for a smoother texture, if desired.

How to Use: Eat this soup when you're menstruating to increase your intake of iron and promote healthy menstruation generally.

Lemon Water Warmed Up for Detoxification

Intended Use: uses lemon water to support the health of the liver and hormones, encouraging cleansing during menstruation.

Ingredients:

- Juice of 1 lemon
- 1 cup warm water

Preparation:

1. Squeeze the lemon juice into a cup of warm water.
2. Stir well to combine.

How to Use: When you are on your period, drink warm lemon water first thing in the morning to promote menstrual health and cleansing.

Apple cider vinegar tonic with cinnamon

Intended Use: Use cinnamon and apple cider vinegar to promote blood sugar balance and relieve menstruation discomfort.

Ingredients:

- 2 tbsp apple cider vinegar
- 1 tsp cinnamon powder
- 1 cup warm water
- Honey to taste (optional)

Preparation:

1. Mix apple cider vinegar and cinnamon powder in warm water.
2. Add honey to taste, if desired, and stir well.

How to Use: For the purpose of reducing menstrual discomfort and promoting general wellbeing, drink this tonic once a day, particularly in the days leading up to and during your period.

HEALTH METALBOLIC

Drink to Boost Metabolism Green Tea with Lemon

Intended Use: uses the purifying qualities of lemon and the antioxidants in green tea to increase metabolic rate and help in fat burning.

Ingredients:

- 1 green tea bag
- Juice of half a lemon
- 1 cup of hot water
- Honey to taste (optional)

Preparation:

1. Steep the green tea bag in hot water for 3-5 minutes.
2. Remove the tea bag and add lemon juice.
3. Sweeten with honey if desired.

How to Use: To increase metabolism, drink one to two cups each day, ideally in the morning and early afternoon.

Ginger-Turmeric Anti-Inflammatory Smoothie

Intended Use: benefits metabolic health and lowers inflammation because to the anti-inflammatory properties of ginger and turmeric.

Ingredients:

- 1 inch fresh turmeric root, peeled (or 1 tsp turmeric powder)
- 1 inch fresh ginger root, peeled
- 1 ripe banana
- ½ cup mango chunks
- 1 cup spinach leaves
- 1 cup almond milk
- A pinch of black pepper (to enhance turmeric absorption)

Preparation:

1. Place all ingredients in a blender.
2. Blend until smooth.
3. Serve immediately for the best taste and nutrient benefits.

How to Use: Drink this smoothie every day to help maintain metabolic health and reduce inflammation.

Apple cider vinegar with cinnamon as a metabolic booster

Intended Use: enhances blood sugar management and metabolism through the use of apple cider vinegar and cinnamon's natural ingredients.

Ingredients:

- 2 tbsp of apple cider vinegar
- 1 tsp of cinnamon powder
- 1 cup of warm water
- Honey to taste (optional)

Preparation:

1. Mix apple cider vinegar and cinnamon powder in warm water.
2. Add honey to taste, if desired, and stir well until combined.
3. Drink this mixture first thing in the morning on an empty stomach.

How to Use: Take once a day to improve blood sugar regulation and metabolic health.

Fermented Vegetable Salad with Probiotics

Intended Use: naturally fermented veggies, high in probiotics, improve intestinal health and metabolism.

Ingredients:

- 1 cup sauerkraut (homemade or store-bought, unpasteurized)
- 1 cup shredded carrots
- ½ cup diced cucumber
- 2 tbsp olive oil
- 1 tbsp apple cider vinegar
- Salt and pepper to taste
- Fresh herbs for garnish (optional)

Preparation:

1. In a large bowl, combine sauerkraut, shredded carrots, and dicedcucumber.
2. Dress with olive oil and apple cider vinegar.
3. Season with salt and pepper to taste.
4. Garnish with fresh herbs if desired.

How to Use: Eat a portion of this salad every day to help maintain healthy digestion and metabolism.

Drink with Spirulina Energy Boost

Intended Use: increases energy and improves metabolic health by using spirulina, a nutrient-dense algae.

Ingredients:

- 1 tsp spirulina powder
- 1 cup coconut water
- Juice of half a lime
- Honey to taste (optional)

Preparation:

1. Mix spirulina powder with coconut water until well dissolved.
2. Add lime juice and honey to taste.
3. Stir well and drink immediately.

How to Use: Indulge in this midmorning or afternoon snack to enhance metabolism and nourish your brain.

Smoothie with Almond Milk and Kale

Intended Use: Containing kale and almond milk, supports metabolism and offers a nutrient-dense start to the day.

Ingredients:

- 2 cups chopped kale leaves
- 1 cup unsweetened almond milk
- 1 banana
- 1 tbsp almond butter

- Ice cubes (optional)

Preparation:

1. Combine kale, almond milk, banana, and almond butter in a blender.
2. Add ice cubes if desired for a chilled smoothie.
3. Blend until smooth.

How to Use: For a healthy snack or breakfast, try this smoothie to help maintain metabolic health.

Brain-Fueling Avocado and Walnut Snack

Intended Use: uses healthy fats from avocado and walnuts to support both metabolic health and cognitive function.

Ingredients:

- 1 ripe avocado, sliced
- ¼ cup walnuts, roughly chopped
- A sprinkle of sea salt
- A drizzle of extra virgin olive oil

Preparation:

1. Arrange avocado slices on a plate.
2. Top with chopped walnuts.
3. Sprinkle with sea salt and drizzle with olive oil.

How to Use: Indulge in this midmorning or afternoon snack to enhance metabolism and nourish your brain.

Chia and Flaxseed Pudding for Digestive Support

Intended Use: fiber-rich flaxseeds and chia seeds promote metabolic health and aid with digestion.

Ingredients:

- 2 tbsp chia seeds
- 1 tbsp ground flaxseeds
- 1 cup almond milk
- 1 tsp vanilla extract

- Berries for topping
- Honey to taste (optional)

Preparation:

1. In a bowl, mix chia seeds, flaxseeds, almond milk, and vanillaextract.
2. Let the mixture sit for at least 30 minutes or overnight in therefrigerator until it forms a pudding-like consistency.
3. Top with berries and honey before serving.

How to Use: Eat this pudding for breakfast or as a dessert to help maintain a healthy metabolism and digestive system.

Dandelion Root Infusion

Intended Use: benefits liver and digestive health by means of dandelion root's cleansing qualities.

Ingredients:

- 1 tbsp dried dandelion root
- 1 cup boiling water

Preparation:

1. Place dandelion root in a tea infuser or directly in a mug.
2. Pour boiling water over the root.
3. Cover and steep for 10 minutes.
4. Strain and drink warm.

How to Use: Drink one to two cups each day, preferably before meals, to help with metabolism and digestive health.

Matcha and Coconut Oil Latte: Boost Your Metabolism

Intended Use: increases energy and metabolism by combining medium-chain triglycerides from coconut oil with antioxidant-rich matcha.

Ingredients:

- 1 tsp matcha green tea powder
- 1 cup hot water
- 1 tbsp coconut oil

- Honey to taste (optional)

Preparation:

1. Whisk matcha powder in hot water until dissolved.
2. Stir in coconut oil until well combined.
3. Sweeten with honey if desired.
4. Froth with a milk frother for a latte effect.

How to Use: Have a drink in the morning to speed up your metabolism and give you energy that lasts all day.

MUSCLE RECOVERY AND GROWTH

Quinoa and Black Bean Salad Packed with Protein

Intended Use: Rich in minerals and amino acids, black beans and high-protein quinoa promote muscular growth and recuperation.

Ingredients:

- 1 cup cooked quinoa
- 1 cup cooked black beans (rinsed if canned)
- 1 avocado, diced
- ½ cup cherry tomatoes, halved
- ¼ cup chopped cilantro
- Juice of 1 lime
- 2 tbsp olive oil
- Salt and pepper to taste

Preparation:

1. In a large bowl, combine the cooked quinoa and black beans.
2. Add the diced avocado, cherry tomatoes, and chopped cilantro.
3. In a small bowl, whisk together lime juice, olive oil, salt, and pepperto create the dressing.
4. Pour the dressing over the salad and gently toss to combine.

How to Use: Savor this salad as a post-workout meal to promote muscular growth and recuperation. It may be eaten at room temperature or chilled.

Berry and Spinach Smoothie

Intended Use: includes protein powder, mixed berries, and spinach to provide nutrients and antioxidants necessary for muscle building and recuperation.

Ingredients:

- 1 cup fresh spinach
- ½ cup mixed berries (fresh or frozen)
- 1 scoop protein powder of choice

- 1 cup almond milk
- 1 tbsp chia seeds

Preparation:

1. Place all ingredients in a blender.
2. Blend on high until smooth.
3. Serve immediately.

How to Use: To optimize muscle growth and recuperation after exercise, drink this smoothie as soon as possible after working out.

Calm Epsom Salt Bath for Your Muscles

Intended Use: Epsom salts' magnesium content relieves pain in the muscles and hastens healing.

Ingredients:

- 2 cups Epsom salt
- 10 drops lavender essential oil (optional for relaxation)
- Warm bath water

Preparation:

1. Fill your bathtub with warm water.
2. Add Epsom salt and lavender essential oil to the bathwater.
3. Stir the water until the salt is dissolved.
4. Soak in the bath for 20-30 minutes.

How to Use: After hard workouts, treat yourself to an Epsom salt bath two or three times a week to promote relaxation and muscle healing.

Ginger and Turmeric Muscle Recovering Tea

Intended Use: uses the anti-inflammatory qualities of turmeric and ginger to reduce inflammation and aid in muscle rehabilitation.

Ingredients:

- 1 inch fresh turmeric root, grated (or 1 tsp turmeric powder)
- 1 inch fresh ginger root, grated
- 1 cup boiling water

- Honey and lemon to taste

Preparation:

1. Place grated turmeric and ginger in a cup.
2. Pour boiling water over the roots and cover.
3. Steep for 10-15 minutes.
4. Strain and add honey and lemon to taste.

How to Use: To promote muscle healing and lessen discomfort, drink one to two cups of it every day, particularly after working out.

Recovering Snack with Sweet Potato and Almond Butter

Intended Use: Supports muscle recovery with complex carbohydrates fromsweet potato and healthy fats and protein from almond butter.

Ingredients:

- 1 medium sweet potato, cooked and sliced
- 2 tbsp almond butter
- Cinnamon to taste

Preparation:

1. Slice the cooked sweet potato.
2. Spread almond butter over the sweet potato slices.
3. Sprinkle with cinnamon.

How to Use: After hard workouts, treat yourself to an Epsom salt bath two or three times a week to promote relaxation and muscle healing.

Rich in Amino Acids Bone Broth

Intended Use: provides nutrient-dense bone broth that provides critical amino acids for muscle development and repair.

Ingredients:

- 2 pounds mixed bones (beef, chicken, or fish)
- 1 onion, quartered
- 2 carrots, chopped
- 2 celery stalks, chopped

- 2 tbsp apple cider vinegar
- Water to cover
- Salt and pepper to taste

Preparation:

1. Place bones in a large pot and cover with water. Add apple cidervinegar.
2. Bring to a boil, then reduce heat and simmer for 12-24 hours, addingwater as necessary.
3. Add vegetables in the last 2 hours of cooking.
4. Strain the broth and season with salt and pepper.

How to Use: Drink one cup of bone broth every day to promote muscle development and regeneration, particularly after exercise.

Avocado, Banana, and Magnesium Pudding

Intended Use: magnesium from bananas and avocados promotes muscular relaxation and healing.

Ingredients:

- 1 ripe banana
- 1 ripe avocado
- 1 tbsp cocoa powder
- Honey or maple syrup to taste

Preparation:

1. Blend banana, avocado, and cocoa powder until smooth.
2. Sweeten with honey or maple syrup to taste.
3. Chill in the refrigerator before serving.

How to Use: Savor this pudding as a dessert or a snack to give your body the nutrition it needs to repair damaged muscles.

Cherry Juice for Pain in the Muscles

Intended Use: uses cherries' inherent anti-inflammatory qualities to lessen muscular discomfort and aid in healing.

Ingredients:

- 1 cup fresh or frozen cherries
- 1 cup water or coconut water
- Honey to taste (optional)

Preparation:

1. Blend cherries and water until smooth.
2. Strain the mixture to remove solids.
3. Sweeten with honey if desired.

How to Use: For faster healing and less stiffness in your muscles after an exercise, try drinking one cup of cherry juice every day.

Herbal Tea for Muscle Relaxation

Intended Use: mix of relaxing herbs that promotes relaxation and eases tense muscles.

Ingredients:

- 1 tsp dried chamomile flowers
- 1 tsp dried lemon balm leaves
- 1 tsp dried valerian root
- 1 cup boiling water

Preparation:

1. Mix chamomile, lemon balm, and valerian root in a tea infuser orteapot.
2. Pour boiling water over the herbs and steep for 10 minutes.
3. Strain and drink warm.

How to Use: Drink this tea in the evening after workouts or before bed tosupport muscle relaxation and recovery.

Greek Yogurt and Hemp Seed Parfait Packed with Protein

Intended Use: provide vital fatty acids and high-quality protein for the development and repair of muscles.

Ingredients:

- 1 cup Greek yogurt
- 2 tbsp hemp seeds
- ½ cup mixed berries

- 1 tbsp honey or maple syrup

Preparation:

1. Layer Greek yogurt, hemp seeds, and mixed berries in a glass orbowl.
2. Drizzle with honey or maple syrup.
3. Repeat layers if desired.

How to Use: Delight in this pudding for dessert or as a snack to provide your body with the nourishment it requires to heal injured muscles.

IMPROVED NUTRIENT ABSORPTION

Probiotic Salad with Fermentation

Intended Use: uses natural probiotics to improve nutrient absorption and digestive health.

Ingredients:

- 1 cup shredded cabbage
- 1 carrot, grated
- 1 beet, grated
- 2 tbsp sea salt
- Water, as needed

Preparation:

1. Combine cabbage, carrot, and beet in a large bowl. Sprinkle with seasalt.
2. Massage the vegetables with your hands until they release theirjuices.
3. Pack the mixture tightly into a jar, leaving at least an inch of space atthe top.
4. Add water to cover the vegetables if they are not fully submerged intheir own liquid.
5. Seal the jar loosely and let it sit at room temperature for 3-7 days forfermentation.
6. Check daily to ensure vegetables are submerged, pressing down ifneeded.

How to Use: Add a tiny portion of this probiotic salad to your meals every day to help maintain intestinal health and enhance the absorption of nutrients.

Smoothie with papaya and pineapple for digestion

Intended Use: Boosts digestion and enzyme production with papain andbromelain.

Ingredients:

- ½ cup ripe papaya, chopped
- ½ cup pineapple, chopped
- 1 cup coconut water
- 1 tsp lime juice
- 1 tbsp honey (optional)

Preparation:

1. Place papaya, pineapple, coconut water, and lime juice in a blender.

2. Blend until smooth.
3. Sweeten with honey if desired.

How to Use: In order to improve the activity of digestive enzymes and the absorption of nutrients, drink this smoothie in the morning on an empty stomach or before to meals.

Tonic with Digestive Bitters

Intended Use: feeds the digestive enzymes to improve the absorption of nutrients.

Ingredients:

- 1 tbsp fresh ginger, grated
- 1 tsp dandelion root
- 1 tsp fennel seeds
- 500ml apple cider vinegar

Preparation:

1. Combine ginger, dandelion root, and fennel seeds in a jar.
2. Pour apple cider vinegar over the herbs, ensuring they are completelysubmerged.
3. Seal the jar and store in a cool, dark place for 2-4 weeks, shakingdaily.
4. After infusion, strain the mixture and store the tonic in a clean bottle.

How to Use: Enjoy this pudding as a snack or dessert to give your body the nutrition it needs to repair damaged muscles.

Digestive Aid Tea with Ginger and Lemon

Intended Use: uses ginger and lemon to improve nutrient absorption and aid with digestion.

Ingredients:

- 1 inch fresh ginger, sliced
- Juice of ½ lemon
- 1 cup boiling water
- Honey (optional)

Preparation:

1. Add ginger slices to a mug and pour boiling water over them.
2. Steep for 5-10 minutes.

3. Add lemon juice and honey to taste.

How to Use: Sip this tea 20 minutes before meals to prepare the digestivesystem for enhanced nutrient absorption.

Drink with Honey and Apple Cider Vinegar

Intended Use: Apple cider vinegar improves stomach acidity and the absorption of nutrients.

Ingredients:

- 1 tbsp apple cider vinegar
- 1 tbsp honey
- 1 cup warm water

Preparation:

1. Dissolve honey in warm water.
2. Add apple cider vinegar and mix well.

How to Use: Drink 15 minutes before meals to increase the amount of acid in your stomach and aid with nutritional absorption.

Digestive Gel with Aloe Vera

Intended Use: Soothes the digestive tract and enhances nutrient absorptionwith aloe vera.

Ingredients:

- 2 tbsp aloe vera gel (freshly extracted or store-bought)
- 1 cup water

Preparation:

1. Blend aloe vera gel with water until smooth.
2. Store the mixture in a sealed container in the refrigerator.

How to Use: On an empty stomach, take 1 tbsp of the aloe vera combination in the morning to promote healthy digestion and nutrient absorption.

Zinc-Rich Pumpkin Seed Pesto

Intended Use: Zinc from pumpkin seeds helps the digestive tract and the body's ability to absorb nutrients.

Ingredients:

- 1 cup fresh basil leaves
- ½ cup pumpkin seeds, toasted
- 2 cloves garlic
- ½ cup olive oil
- Salt and pepper to taste

Preparation:

1. Combine basil, pumpkin seeds, and garlic in a food processor andpulse until coarsely chopped.
2. With the processor running, gradually add olive oil until the mixtureis smooth.
3. Season with salt and pepper.

How to Use: Use this pesto as a sandwich spread or pasta sauce to get zinc into your diet for better digestive health.

Nutrient-Enhancing Herbal Broth

Intended Use: gives a foundation for nutrient absorption with a combination of herbs that aid in digestion.

Ingredients:

- 4 cups water
- 1 onion, chopped
- 2 carrots, chopped
- 2 celery stalks, chopped
- 1 tbsp turmeric root, grated
- 1 tbsp ginger root, grated
- 1 tsp black pepper
- 1 tsp sea salt

Preparation:

1. Combine all ingredients in a large pot.

2. Bring to a boil, then simmer for 1 hour.
3. Strain the broth and discard the solids.

How to Use: To improve nutrient absorption, have a cup of herbal broth half an hour before meals or use it as the foundation for soups and stews.

Water with Lemon and Flaxseed

Intended Use: fiber from flaxseeds encourages a healthy digestive system and the absorption of nutrients.

Ingredients:

- 1 tbsp ground flaxseed
- Juice of 1 lemon
- 1 cup warm water

Preparation:

1. Stir ground flaxseed and lemon juice into warm water.
2. Let sit for 5 minutes before drinking.

How to Use: To improve nutrient absorption, have a cup of herbal broth half an hour before meals or use it as the foundation for soups and stews.

Peppermint and Fennel Seed Digestive Tea

Intended Use: uses fennel and peppermint to improve nutrition absorption and ease stomach pain.

Ingredients:

- 1 tsp dried peppermint leaves
- 1 tsp fennel seeds
- 1 cup boiling water

Preparation:

1. Crush fennel seeds slightly to release their oil.
2. Place peppermint leaves and fennel seeds in a cup or tea infuser.
3. Pour boiling water over the herbs and cover.
4. Steep for 10 minutes, then strain.

How to Use: To improve nutrition absorption and assist with digestion, sip this tea after meals.

HEALTH OF RESPIRATORY SYSTEM

Inhaling Steam Eucalyptus

Intended Use: Because of eucalyptus's decongestant qualities, it helps to clear respiratory airways and relieve breathing troubles.

Ingredients:

- 3-5 drops of eucalyptus essential oil
- A bowl of boiling water

Preparation:

1. Add eucalyptus essential oil to the bowl of boiling water.
2. Lean over the bowl and cover your head with a towel to trap thesteam.
3. Inhale the steam deeply for 5-10 minutes.

How to Use: Once or twice a day, especially if you have congestion or respiratory pain, perform this inhalation.

Tea with Mullein Leaf

Intended Use: thanks to mullein's expectorant qualities, supports lung health and helps the respiratory system rid itself of mucus.

Ingredients:

- 1-2 tsps dried mullein leaves
- 1 cup boiling water

Preparation:

1. Place mullein leaves in a cup or tea infuser.
2. Pour boiling water over the leaves and steep for 10 minutes.
3. Strain and drink the tea warm.

How to Use: Drink 2-3 cups daily to support respiratory health.

Anti-inflammatory drink with ginger and turmeric.

Intended Use: reduces respiratory system irritation by using the anti-inflammatory qualities of turmeric and ginger.

Ingredients:

- 1 inch fresh ginger, grated
- 1 tsp turmeric powder
- Juice of 1 lemon
- 1 tbsp honey
- 2 cups hot water

Preparation:

1. Add ginger, turmeric, and hot water to a pot and simmer for 10minutes.
2. Strain the mixture into a cup, add lemon juice and honey.
3. Stir well and drink warm.

How to Use: Eat once or twice a day to assist in lowering inflammation in the respiratory system.

Honey-Thyme Cough Syrup

Intended Use: Because thyme and honey have antibacterial qualities, they help to soothe coughs and sore throats while promoting respiratory health.

Ingredients:

- ¼ cup fresh thyme leaves
- 1 cup water
- 1 cup honey

Preparation:

1. Boil water and add thyme leaves. Simmer for 15 minutes.
2. Strain the thyme leaves and mix the thyme-infused water with honeyin a saucepan.
3. Heat gently until well combined, then allow to cool beforetransferring to a glass jar.

How to Use: Take 1 tbsp whenever you need to relieve a cough.

Tea with peppermint and licorice root

Intended Use: Peppermint soothes the throat and opens the airways, and licorice root soothes inflammation by acting as a demulcent.

Ingredients:

- 1 tsp dried peppermint leaves
- 1 tsp dried licorice root
- 1 cup boiling water

Preparation:

1. Mix peppermint leaves and licorice root in a cup or tea infuser.
2. Pour boiling water over the herbs and steep for 10 minutes.
3. Strain and drink the tea warm.

How to Use: Up to two cups of liquids should be consumed each day, particularly if you have lung or throat irritation.

Sweet Potato and Onion Respiratory Tonic

Intended Use: Offers antimicrobial and expectorant properties to supportrespiratory health and ease coughs.

Ingredients:

- 1 medium onion, finely chopped
- ½ cup honey

Preparation:

1. Combine onion and honey in a bowl. Cover and let sit for 12 hours.
2. Strain the mixture, pressing the onion to extract all liquid.
3. Store the liquid (tonic) in a glass jar.

How to Use: Take 1 tbsp of the tonic as needed for respiratory support and cough alleviation every few hours.

Pine Needle Cough Drops

Intended Use: Pine needles' antibacterial qualities and vitamin C soothe coughs and promote respiratory health.

Ingredients:

- ½ cup chopped pine needles (from a safe, edible variety)
- 1 cup water
- 1 cup sugar

- 1 tbsp honey
- 1 tbsp lemon juice

Preparation:

1. Boil pine needles in water for 20 minutes. Strain and reserve the liquid.
2. In a saucepan, combine the pine needle liquid, sugar, honey, and lemon juice. Heat until the mixture reaches the hard-crack stage(300°F).
3. Pour the mixture into molds or drop by spoonfuls onto a parchment- lined tray.
4. Allow to cool and harden before using.

How to Use: To relieve a cough, dissolve one cough drop in your mouth as needed.

Aromatherapy Chest Rub

Intended Use: A combination of essential oils that support healthy breathing helps to relieve respiratory irritation and promotes clean breathing.

Ingredients:

- 2 tbsp coconut oil
- 4 drops eucalyptus essential oil
- 4 drops peppermint essential oil
- 2 drops thyme essential oil

Preparation:

1. Gently melt the coconut oil in a small container.
2. Add the essential oils to the melted coconut oil and stir to combine.
3. Allow the mixture to solidify.

How to Use: To maintain respiratory health, rub a tiny quantity on the back and chest two to three times a day, especially right before bed.

Smoothie with Sea Moss Respiratory

Intended Use: uses sea moss's mucilage and nutrient-rich qualities to improve respiratory health.

Ingredients:

- 2 tbsp sea moss gel
- 1 cup almond milk

- ½ banana
- ½ cup mango chunks
- 1 tsp honey

Preparation:

1. Blend sea moss gel, almond milk, banana, and mango chunks untilsmooth.
2. Sweeten with honey to taste.

How to Use: Drink this smoothie every day to help your immune system and respiratory system stay healthy.

Herbal Lung-Cleansing Inhaler

Intended Use: combines a combination of purifying herbs to support respiratory system cleaning and detoxification.

Ingredients:

- 1 tsp dried mullein
- 1 tsp dried peppermint
- 1 tsp dried eucalyptus
- Aromatherapy inhaler tube

Preparation:

1. Finely grind the dried herbs and mix together.
2. Open the aromatherapy inhaler tube and pack the ground herb mixture into the refillable section according to the manufacturer's instructions.
3. Close the inhaler securely.

How to Use: Take three to four deep breaths from the inhaler each day, especially if you're having trouble breathing or just want to regularly maintain the health of your lungs. Mullein, peppermint, and eucalyptus work in concert to assist the lungs' natural detoxifying processes, ease respiratory tract irritation, and encourage easy breathing.

IMPROVED RESPIRATORY SYSTEM

Lung Cleansing Herbal Tea

Intended Use: mix of herbs known to be effective lung cleaners to support respiratory health and remove congestion.

Ingredients:

- 1 tsp mullein leaf
- 1 tsp peppermint leaf
- 1 tsp licorice root
- 2 cups boiling water

Preparation:

1. Combine mullein, peppermint, and licorice root in a teapot or largemug.
2. Pour boiling water over the herbs and steep for 10 minutes.
3. Strain and enjoy the tea warm.

How to Use: Sip one to two glasses every day to help maintain respiratory health and reduce congestion.

Healthy Bone Broth

Intended Use: provide vital nutrients that support a healthy immune system and respiratory system in general.

Ingredients:

- 2 pounds mixed bones (chicken, beef, or fish)
- 2 carrots, chopped
- 2 celery stalks, chopped
- 1 onion, chopped
- 2 tbsp apple cider vinegar
- Water to cover
- Salt and pepper to taste

Preparation:

1. Place all ingredients in a large pot or slow cooker.
2. Add enough water to cover the bones and vegetables.
3. Bring to a boil, then reduce heat and simmer for 24-48 hours,skimming off any foam that forms.
4. Strain the broth and season with salt and pepper.
5. Store in the refrigerator or freezer for later use.

How to Use: Use one cup of bone broth as a foundation for soups and stews or consume it as a nutritious beverage once a day.

Elderberry Syrup to Boost Immunity

Intended Use: elderberries, which are high in antioxidants, strengthen the respiratory system and enhance the immunological response.

Ingredients:

- ½ cup dried elderberries
- 3 cups water
- 1 cinnamon stick
- 5 cloves
- 1 piece of fresh ginger, sliced
- 1 cup honey

Preparation:

1. Combine elderberries, water, cinnamon, cloves, and ginger in asaucepan.
2. Bring to a boil, reduce heat, and simmer for 45 minutes to an houruntil the liquid has reduced by half.
3. Remove from heat, cool, and strain the liquid.
4. Stir in honey until well combined.
5. Store in a glass bottle in the refrigerator.

How to Use: During the cold and flu season, use 1 tbsp daily to support a stronger immune system and respiratory system.

Eucalyptus and Peppermint Chest Rub

Intended Use: opens airways and facilitates breathing by using the decongestant qualities of eucalyptus and peppermint.

Ingredients:

- ¼ cup coconut oil
- 10 drops peppermint essential oil
- 10 drops eucalyptus essential oil

Preparation:

1. Melt coconut oil in a double boiler or microwave.
2. Remove from heat and stir in peppermint and eucalyptus essentialoils.
3. Pour the mixture into a small jar and let it solidify.

How to Use: Apply a tiny quantity to the back and chest as needed, especially right before bed, to facilitate breathing and open up respiratory channels.

Immune Booster with Oregano Oil

Intended Use: uses oregano oil's antibacterial qualities to fight infections and strengthen the respiratory system.

Ingredients:

- 1 drop oregano essential oil
- 1 tbsp olive oil or coconut oil

Preparation:

1. Mix oregano oil with olive or coconut oil in a small bowl.
2. Store in a glass bottle.

How to Use: Once a day, use a little quantity of the diluted oregano oil combination on the spine or beneath the feet to promote respiratory health and strengthen the immune system.

Root of Astragalus Immune Tonic

Intended Use: Enhances respiratory health and immune function with theadaptogenic properties of astragalus root.

Ingredients:

- 1 tbsp dried astragalus root
- 4 cups water

Preparation:

1. Combine astragalus root and water in a saucepan.
2. Bring to a boil, then simmer for 30 minutes.
3. Strain and consume the tonic warm or cold.

How to Use: Astragalus tonic should be consumed once a day to promote respiratory and immunological health.

Sea Moss Gel to Assist with Respiration

Intended Use: gives the respiratory system the minerals and nutrients it needs by using the mucilaginous qualities of sea moss.

Ingredients:

- ½ cup dried sea moss
- 2 cups filtered water
- Additional water for blending

Preparation:

1. Rinse sea moss thoroughly and soak in 2 cups of water for 12-24hours.
2. Drain and rinse again, then blend with just enough fresh water tocreate a gel.
3. Store the gel in a sealed container in the refrigerator.

How to Use: With meals, take one or two capsules daily to promote lung health and lower inflammation.

Honey-Lemon Respiratory Tea

Intended Use: With the antibacterial qualities of honey and the vitamin C in lemon, it soothes the throat and promotes respiratory health.

Ingredients:

- Juice of 1 lemon
- 1 tbsp raw honey
- 1 cup hot water

Preparation:

1. Stir lemon juice and honey into hot water until well combined.
2. Drink warm.

How to Use: With meals, take one or two capsules daily to promote lung health and lower inflammation.

Black pepper and turmeric lung health capsules

Intended Use: reduces inflammation and promotes respiratory health by utilizing black pepper to increase the anti-inflammatory qualities of turmeric.

Ingredients:

- 1 part turmeric powder
- ¼ part ground black pepper
- Empty capsules

Preparation:

1. Mix turmeric powder and black pepper thoroughly.
2. Fill empty capsules with the mixture using a capsule filling machineor a small spoon.
3. Store in a cool, dry place.

How to Use: With meals, take one or two capsules daily to promote lung health and lower inflammation.

Thyme Antiseptic Inhalation Spray

Intended Use: Supports respiratory health and clears airways with the antiseptic properties of thyme.

Ingredients:

- 1 tbsp dried thyme
- 1 bowl of boiling water

Preparation:

1. Add dried thyme to a bowl of boiling water.
2. Lean over the bowl and cover your head with a towel to trap thesteam.
3. Inhale the steam for 5-10 minutes, taking care not to get too close tothe hot water.

How to Use: As required, use this inhalant one to two times a day to help maintain respiratory health and reduce congestion.

HAIR AND SKIN NUTRITION

Honey and Aloe Vera Face Mask

Intended Use: Aloe vera and honey's natural characteristics are used to moisturize and cure the skin.

Ingredients:

- 2 tbsp aloe vera gel
- 1 tbsp raw honey

Preparation:

1. Mix aloe vera gel and raw honey in a small bowl until wellcombined.
2. Apply the mixture to a clean face and leave on for 20 minutes.
3. Rinse off with warm water and pat dry.

How to Use: Use 2-3 times a week for hydrated, glowing skin.

Green Tea Skin Toner

Intended Use: uses green tea's antioxidants to tighten pores and reduce irritation.

Ingredients:

- 1 cup water
- 2 green tea bags

Preparation:

1. Boil water and steep green tea bags for 15 minutes.
2. Remove tea bags and allow the tea to cool to room temperature.
3. Pour the green tea into a clean bottle.

How to Use: Use a cotton ball to apply on the face in the morning and evening after cleaning.

Egg and Avocado Hair Mask

Intended Use: The nutritious fats in avocado and the protein in eggs help to restore moisture and vitality to dry or damaged hair.

Ingredients:

- 1 ripe avocado
- 1 egg

Preparation:

1. Mash the avocado in a bowl.
2. Beat the egg and mix it with the avocado until smooth.
3. Apply to damp hair, covering from roots to tips.
4. Leave on for 20 minutes, then rinse and shampoo as usual.

How to Use: For optimal results in repairing and moisturizing hair, use once every two weeks.

Hair Treatment with Coconut Oil

Intended Use: Coconut oil fortifies and nourishes hair, encouraging growth and averting damage.

Ingredients:

- 3 tbsp coconut oil (melted)
- 1 tbsp olive oil

Preparation:

1. Mix coconut oil and olive oil in a bowl.
2. Apply the mixture to your hair, focusing on the ends and avoiding
3. the scalp if prone to oiliness.
4. Leave on for at least 30 minutes or overnight for deep conditioning.
5. Wash hair as usual.

How to Use: For optimal results in terms of hair strength and shine, use once a week.

Yogurt and Oatmeal Calming Face Scrub

Intended Use: uses yogurt and oatmeal's natural qualities to gently exfoliate and soothe skin.

Ingredients:

- 2 tbsp ground oatmeal
- 2 tbsp plain yogurt

- 1 tsp honey

Preparation:

1. Combine all ingredients in a bowl to form a paste.
2. Gently massage onto the face in circular motions, avoiding the eyearea.
3. Rinse off with warm water.

How to Use: Once a week, use to get soft, exfoliated skin.

Herbal Shine Hair Rinse

Intended Use: improves scalp health and hair gloss with a combination of nutritious herbs.

Ingredients:

- 2 tbsp dried rosemary
- 2 tbsp dried nettle
- 1 quart water

Preparation:

1. Boil water and add herbs.
2. Simmer for 15 minutes, then let cool.
3. Strain the mixture and pour into a container.

How to Use: After shampooing, use as a last rinse; do not rinse out. Apply up to twice a week to ensure healthy, lustrous hair.

Mint and Cucumber Eye Gel

Intended Use: Reduces puffiness and dark circles under the eyes with thesoothing properties of cucumber and mint.

Ingredients:

- ½ cucumber
- ¼ cup fresh mint leaves
- 1 tbsp aloe vera gel

Preparation:

1. Blend cucumber and mint leaves until smooth.

2. Strain the mixture to extract the juice.
3. Mix the juice with aloe vera gel and store in a small jar.

How to Use: Before going to bed at night, apply softly around the eyes. To get even more cooling, store in the refrigerator.

Rosehip Oil Night Serum

Intended Use: Rosehip oil's inherent vitamins and fatty acids help to hydrate the skin and lessen the appearance of age.

Ingredients:

- 2 tbsp rosehip oil
- 1 tbsp jojoba oil
- 2 drops lavender essential oil

Preparation:

1. Mix all oils in a small bottle.
2. Shake well to combine.

How to Use: After cleaning, apply a few drops to the face and neck before going to bed.

Lavender and Chamomile Aromatherapy Oil for Sleepy Scalp

Intended Use: provides a calming scalp massage that encourages relaxation and aids in hair development.

Ingredients:

- 2 tbsp sweet almond oil
- 5 drops lavender essential oil
- 5 drops chamomile essential oil

Preparation:

1. Mix all oils in a small bottle and shake well to blend.
2. Warm the oil slightly by placing the bottle in warm water.

How to Use: Before going to bed, give your scalp a 10-minute massage to help you unwind and feed the roots of your hair.

Body Scrub with Exfoliating Sesame Seeds

Intended Use: The nutritious oils in sesame seeds exfoliate and hydrate the skin.

Ingredients:

- ½ cup ground sesame seeds
- ¼ cup sesame oil
- ¼ cup brown sugar

Preparation:

1. Mix ground sesame seeds, sesame oil, and brown sugar in a bowluntil well combined.
2. Apply to wet skin in the shower, massaging in circular motions.
3. Rinse off thoroughly with warm water.

How to Use: Use once a week to remove dead skin cells and moisturize theskin deeply.

STRESS MANAGEMENT

Smoothie with Adaptogen Stress Relief

Intended Use: Adaptogenic herbs enhance energy levels and support the body's reaction to stress.

Ingredients:

- 1 banana
- 1 cup spinach
- 1 tbsp ashwagandha powder
- 1 tbsp maca powder
- 1 cup almond milk
- A handful of blueberries

Preparation:

1. Place all ingredients in a blender.
2. Blend on high until smooth.
3. Serve immediately.

How to Use: Take in the morning or when you're feeling stressed to help with energy and stress relief.

Herbal Infusion of Holy Basil (Tulsi)

Intended Use: because holy basil has adaptogenic properties that help reduce stress and anxiety.

Ingredients:

- 2 tbsp dried holy basil leaves (Tulsi)
- 1 quart boiling water

Preparation:

1. Place holy basil leaves in a large jar.
2. Pour boiling water over the leaves and cover.
3. Let the infusion steep for at least 4 hours or overnight.
4. Strain and refrigerate.

How to Use: Have a glass of the infusion every day to help elevate your mood and reduce stress.

Calming Tea with Chamomile and Lavender

Intended Use: has calming effects on the neurological system and lowers stress levels thanks to lavender and chamomile.

Ingredients:

- 1 tsp dried chamomile flowers
- ½ tsp dried lavender buds
- 1 cup boiling water
- Honey (optional)

Preparation:

1. Combine chamomile and lavender in a tea infuser or teapot.
2. Pour boiling water over the herbs and cover.
3. Steep for 5-10 minutes, depending on desired strength.
4. Strain into a mug and sweeten with honey if desired.

How to Use: Drink in the evening or whenever stress levels are high to promote relaxation and reduce anxiety.

Essential Oil Stress Relief Roller

Intended Use: use a combination of relaxing essential oils to provide instantaneous stress relief and relaxation.

Ingredients:

- 10 ml carrier oil (jojoba, sweet almond, or coconut oil)
- 4 drops lavender essential oil
- 3 drops frankincense essential oil
- 3 drops bergamot essential oil
- Roller bottle

Preparation:

1. Add essential oils to the roller bottle.
2. Fill the rest of the bottle with the carrier oil.

3. Cap the bottle and shake well to mix.

How to Use: Apply to wrists, temples, and the area behind the ears (pulse points) anytime you feel anxious.

Bath Soak for Relieving Stress

Intended Use: A calming bath soak helps to calm the body and mind and reduce stress on both the physical and mental levels.

Ingredients:

- 1 cup Epsom salts
- ½ cup baking soda
- 10 drops lavender essential oil
- 5 drops chamomile essential oil

Preparation:

1. Mix Epsom salts and baking soda in a bowl.
2. Add essential oils and stir to combine.
3. Store in an airtight container.

How to Use: To reduce stress, add ¼ to ½ cup of the bath soak to warm bath water and soak for at least 20 minutes.

Focus Spray with Peppermint and Rosemary

Intended Use: Reduces stress and increases focus and mental clarity with arefreshing herbal spray.

Ingredients:

- 1 cup distilled water
- 5 drops peppermint essential oil
- 5 drops rosemary essential oil
- Spray bottle

Preparation:

1. Fill the spray bottle with distilled water.
2. Add peppermint and rosemary essential oils.
3. Shake well to mix.

How to Use: When you need a mental lift or stress alleviation, scatter this around your house or place of business.

Ginger and Ginseng Tonic for Optimum Health

Intended Use: Ginseng and ginger are used to improve energy levels, both mental and physical, and stress tolerance.

Ingredients:

- 1 inch fresh ginger root, thinly sliced
- 1 tsp dried ginseng root
- 2 cups water
- Honey to taste

Preparation:

1. Combine ginger, ginseng, and water in a small saucepan.
2. Bring to a boil, then simmer for 20 minutes.
3. Strain into a mug and add honey to taste.

How to Use: Drink every morning to help reduce stress and boost your energy.

Drink with Cacao and Almonds to Boost Mood

Intended Use: Enhances mood and lessens stress because to cacao's inherent ability to elevate mood.

Ingredients:

- 2 tbsp raw cacao powder
- 1 tbsp almond butter
- 1 cup warm almond milk
- Honey or maple syrup to taste

Preparation:

1. Whisk cacao powder and almond butter into warm almond milk untilsmooth.
2. Sweeten with honey or maple syrup to taste.

How to Use: Sip this beverage in the afternoon or anytime you want to decompress and relieve tension.

Nighttime Tea with Valerian Root and Lemon Balm

Intended Use: combines valerian root and lemon balm to encourage sound sleep and lessen tension at night.

Ingredients:

- 1 tsp dried lemon balm leaves
- ½ tsp dried valerian root
- 1 cup boiling water

Preparation:

1. Combine lemon balm and valerian root in a tea infuser or teapot.
2. Pour boiling water over the herbs and steep for 10 minutes.
3. Strain into a mug and drink warm.

How to Use: Thirty minutes before bed, have a drink to lower tension and enhance sleep quality.

Stress-Reduction Candle with Aromatherapy

Intended Use: uses the healing properties of essential oils to create a peaceful environment and reduce stress.

Ingredients:

- Natural soy wax or beeswax
- Wick
- 10 drops lavender essential oil
- 5 drops ylang-ylang essential oil
- Candle mold or container

Preparation:

1. Melt the wax in a double boiler.
2. Once melted, remove from heat and add essential oils, stirring well.
3. Place the wick in the center of the mold or container.
4. Pour the wax into the mold and let it cool and harden.
5. Trim the wick to about ½ inch above the wax.

How to Use: Light the candle during periods of stress or in the evening torelax and unwind.

RELIEF FROM STRESS

Stress-Relieving Tea with Licorice Root and Ashwagandha

Intended Use: uses licorice root's calming effects and ashwagandha's adaptogenic qualities to combat stress and adrenal exhaustion.

Ingredients:

- 1 tsp ashwagandha powder
- 1 tsp licorice root
- 2 cups of water
- Honey or lemon to taste (optional)

Preparation:

1. Add ashwagandha powder and licorice root to water in a saucepan.
2. Bring to a boil, then simmer for 15 minutes.
3. Strain the tea into a mug, adding honey or lemon if desired.
4. Enjoy warm.

How to Use: Drink once daily, preferably in the evening, to help unwind andmanage stress levels.

Chamomile and Mint Relaxation Bath Soak

Intended Use: A soothing bath soak infused with chamomile and mint calms the nervous system and promotes physical relaxation.

Ingredients:

- ½ cup dried chamomile flowers
- ½ cup dried mint leaves
- 1 cup Epsom salts

Preparation:

1. Mix chamomile, mint, and Epsom salts in a bowl.
2. Store the mixture in an airtight container.
3. To use, add 1 cup of the mixture to a warm bath.

How to Use: Take a 20–30 minute soak to decompress and relieve tension.

Tulsi (holy basil) Infused Honey

Intended Use: increases the ability of the body and mind to withstand stress thanks to the adaptogenic properties of holy basil incorporated in honey.

Ingredients:

- 1 cup raw honey
- 2 tbsp dried holy basil leaves (Tulsi)

Preparation:

1. Warm honey in a double boiler until it becomes liquid.
2. Add holy basil leaves and stir gently.
3. Remove from heat and let the mixture infuse for 24-48 hours.
4. Strain the honey into a clean jar, removing all leaves.

How to Use: To help lower stress levels, add a spoonful of this infused honey to a daily cup of tea or warm water.

Stress Relieving Roller with Lavender Essential Oil

Intended Use: instantly reduces tension and encourages rest thanks to lavender essential oil's soothing aroma.

Ingredients:

- 10 ml carrier oil (jojoba or almond oil)
- 7 drops lavender essential oil
- Roller bottle

Preparation:

1. Fill the roller bottle with the carrier oil.
2. Add lavender essential oil to the carrier oil.
3. Cap the bottle and shake well to blend the oils.
4. Label the bottle for easy identification.

How to Use: Roll onto pulse points such as wrists, temples, and behind theears when feeling stressed or anxious.

Tea with Ginseng and Jujube

Intended Use: uses the reviving qualities of ginseng and the soothing effects of jujube to boost energy and relieve stress.

Ingredients:

- 1-inch piece of ginseng root, sliced
- 5 dried jujube fruits
- 4 cups of water

Preparation:

1. Place ginseng slices and jujube fruits in a pot with water.
2. Bring to a boil, then simmer for 20 minutes.
3. Strain and serve the tea warm.

How to Use: Have a drink in the morning or early afternoon to boost resistance to stress and energy.

Herbal Pillow Spray for Stress Reduction

Intended Use: enhances sleep quality and relaxation by diffusing a soothing aroma with the use of a herbal pillow spray.

Ingredients:

- 1 cup distilled water
- 10 drops lavender essential oil
- 5 drops chamomile essential oil
- 5 drops vetiver essential oil
- Spray bottle

Preparation:

1. Fill the spray bottle with distilled water.
2. Add the lavender, chamomile, and vetiver essential oils to the water.
3. Cap the bottle and shake well to ensure the oils are well mixed with the water.
4. Label the bottle for future reference.

How to Use: Before retiring to bed, lightly mist your pillow and sheets with the herbal spray. Use on a regular basis to help lower stress and enhance sleep quality.

Adaptogen-Packed Stress Relief Smoothie

Intended Use: Smoothie rich in nutrients that contains adaptogenic herbs to boost adrenal function and fight stress.

Ingredients:

- 1 cup almond milk
- ½ banana
- ½ cup mixed berries (blueberries, strawberries, raspberries)
- 1 tbsp ashwagandha powder
- 1 tsp rhodiola powder
- 1 tbsp flaxseed meal
- Honey or maple syrup, to taste

Preparation:

1. Add all ingredients to a blender.
2. Blend on high until smooth and creamy.
3. Taste and adjust sweetness with honey or maple syrup if needed.

How to Use: Consume this smoothie in the morning or when you're under a lot of stress to help your body become more resilient and less tired.

Peppermint Balm for Pain Relief

Intended Use: Alleviates headaches and reduces stress with the cooling andsoothing effects of peppermint.

Ingredients:

- 2 tbsp coconut oil
- 1 tbsp beeswax pellets
- 12 drops peppermint essential oil

Preparation:

1. Melt coconut oil and beeswax together in a double boiler.
2. Remove from heat and stir in peppermint essential oil.
3. Pour into a small container and let it solidify.

How to Use: When under stress or having a headache, apply to the back of the neck and the temples.

Stress-Reduction Water Infusion with Rosemary and Lemon

Intended Use: Hydrating blend of lemon and rosemary, recognized for their mood-boosting qualities, refreshes and eases tension.

Ingredients:

- 1 liter of water
- 1 lemon, thinly sliced
- 2 sprigs of fresh rosemary

Preparation:

1. Fill a pitcher with water.
2. Add the sliced lemon and rosemary sprigs to the water.
3. Refrigerate for at least 2 hours, allowing the flavors to infuse.
4. Serve chilled.

How to Use: In order to keep hydrated and lower your stress levels, drink throughout the day.

Cacao and Maca Stress Relief Balls

Intended Use: uses maca powder and cacao to create a nutritious, uplifting snack that can aid with stress management and mood enhancement.

Ingredients:

- 1 cup dates, pitted
- ½ cup raw almonds
- ¼ cup raw cacao powder
- 2 tbsp maca powder
- 1 tbsp coconut oil
- Shredded coconut, for coating

Preparation:

1. In a food processor, blend the dates and almonds until they form asticky mixture.
2. Add the cacao powder, maca powder, and coconut oil to the mixture.Process again

until well combined.

3. Take small amounts of the mixture and roll into balls.
4. Roll the balls in shredded coconut to coat.
5. Place in the refrigerator for at least 30 minutes to set.

How to Use: When you need an energy boost or are feeling worried, eat one or two cacao and maca stress relief balls as a nutritious snack.

SUPPORT FOR THYROID FUNCTION

Mix of Brazil Nuts Thyroid Snacks

Intended Use: Brazil nuts provide selenium, which is essential for thyroid function.

Ingredients:

- 1 cup Brazil nuts
- ½ cup sunflower seeds
- ½ cup pumpkin seeds
- 1 tbsp coconut oil, melted
- A pinch of sea salt

Preparation:

1. Preheat oven to 350°F (175°C).
2. Mix Brazil nuts, sunflower seeds, and pumpkin seeds in a bowl.
3. Add melted coconut oil and sea salt. Stir to coat.
4. Spread the mix on a baking sheet and bake for 10-12 minutes.
5. Let cool before serving.

How to Use: Enjoy a small handful daily to boost selenium intake for thyroidsupport.

Healthy Green Smoothie for the Thyroid

Intended Use: Supports overall thyroid function with nutrient-rich greensand fruits.

Ingredients:

- 1 cup spinach
- 1 cup kale
- 1 banana
- ½ cup blueberries
- 1 tbsp chia seeds
- 1 cup water or almond milk

Preparation:

1. Place all ingredients in a blender.

2. Blend until smooth.
3. Serve immediately.

How to Use: For optimal thyroid health and energy levels, drink this smoothie every day, preferably first thing in the morning.

Salad with Seaweed and Cucumber to Boost Thyroid

Intended Use: uses cucumber's moisturizing qualities and seaweed's natural iodine to support thyroid function.

Ingredients:

- 1 cup fresh seaweed (e.g., arame, wakame), soaked and drained
- 1 cucumber, thinly sliced
- 1 tbsp sesame oil
- 2 tbsp rice vinegar
- 1 tsp honey
- Sesame seeds for garnish

Preparation:

1. Combine seaweed and cucumber in a mixing bowl.
2. In a small bowl, whisk together sesame oil, rice vinegar, and honey.
3. Pour dressing over seaweed and cucumber. Toss to coat.
4. Sprinkle sesame seeds on top before serving.

How to Use: Consume this salad frequently—at least twice or three times a week—to enhance your natural iodine intake and promote thyroid function.

Herbal Ashwagandha Tea

Intended Use: uses ashwagandha to boost thyroid function and reduce stress.

Ingredients:

- 1 tsp ashwagandha powder
- 1 cup boiling water
- Honey or lemon to taste (optional)

Preparation:

1. Add ashwagandha powder to a cup.

2. Pour boiling water over the powder and stir.
3. Steep for 5-7 minutes.
4. Add honey or lemon to taste, if desired.

How to Use: Drink once a day to help thyroid health and regulate stress, ideally in the evening.

Ginger and Turmeric Tea for Thyroid Support

Intended Use: uses ginger and turmeric to help boost thyroid function and reduce inflammation.

Ingredients:

- 1 inch fresh turmeric root, grated
- 1 inch fresh ginger root, grated
- 2 cups water
- Honey to taste

Preparation:

1. Add turmeric and ginger to water in a pot.
2. Bring to a boil, then simmer for 10 minutes.
3. Strain into a mug.
4. Add honey to taste.

How to Use: Drink 1-2 cups daily to support thyroid health and reduceinflammation.

Almond and Flaxseed Porridge for Thyroid Health

Intended Use: high omega-3 content in flaxseed and selenium in almonds support thyroid function.

Ingredients:

- ½ cup ground flaxseed
- ¼ cup sliced almonds
- 1 cup almond milk
- 1 tsp cinnamon
- Honey or maple syrup to taste

Preparation:

1. Heat almond milk in a saucepan over medium heat.
2. Add ground flaxseed and cinnamon, stirring continuously untilthickened.
3. Transfer to a bowl and top with sliced almonds.
4. Sweeten with honey or maple syrup as desired.

How to Use: To promote thyroid function, eat many times each week during breakfast.

Bowl of Kelp Noodle Thyroid Boost

Intended Use: uses kelp noodles to boost iodine consumption for thyroid support.

Ingredients:

- 2 cups kelp noodles, rinsed
- 1 cup shredded carrots
- 1 cup sliced red bell pepper
- 1 avocado, sliced
- ¼ cup tamari sauce
- 1 tbsp sesame oil
- 1 tbsp rice vinegar
- 1 tsp grated ginger

Preparation:

1. Combine kelp noodles, carrots, and red bell pepper in a bowl.
2. In a separate bowl, whisk together tamari sauce, sesame oil, ricevinegar, and ginger.
3. Pour the dressing over the noodle mixture and toss to coat.
4. Top with sliced avocado.

How to Use: For thyroid support, include this dish in your diet two or three times a week.

Selenium-Rich Mixed Nut Butter

Intended Use: provides important nutrients through a combination of nuts, including selenium, for thyroid health.

Ingredients:

- 1 cup Brazil nuts
- ½ cup walnuts

- ½ cup cashews
- 1-2 tbsp coconut oil
- A pinch of sea salt

Preparation:

1. Preheat oven to 350°F (175°C) and roast nuts for 8-10 minutes.
2. Allow nuts to cool, then blend in a food processor, adding coconutoil to achieve desired consistency.
3. Season with sea salt.
4. Store in an airtight container in the refrigerator.

How to Use: Increase your intake of selenium for thyroid health by using it as a spread on whole-grain toast or adding it to smoothies.

Ginger-Dandelion Detox Tea

Intended Use: improves hormone metabolism, which obliquely benefits thyroid health by supporting liver detoxification.

Ingredients:

- 1 tbsp dandelion root (dried)
- 2 cups water
- Lemon slice and honey to taste

Preparation:

1. Boil water and add dandelion root.
2. Simmer for 10 minutes, then strain.
3. Serve with lemon and honey to taste.

How to Use: Drink once a day, either in the morning or right before meals, to help with thyroid health and detoxification.

Enhancer of Spirulina Energy

Intended Use: Enhances thyroid function and overall vitality with thenutrient-rich algae, spirulina.

Ingredients:

- 1 tsp spirulina powder

- 1 cup coconut water
- ½ banana
- ½ cup fresh spinach
- Juice of ½ lime

Preparation:

1. Place all ingredients in a blender.
2. Blend until smooth.
3. Serve immediately.

How to Use: Drink this spirulina-infused beverage in the morning or before workouts to boost energy and support thyroid function with its high iodine content.

CLEANSE AND DETOX THE BODY

Ginger and Lemon Detox Water

Intended Use: benefits from the anti-inflammatory qualities of ginger and the vitamin C of lemon to aid with digestion and detoxification while also having a cleaning impact.

Ingredients:

- 1 liter of water
- 1 lemon, thinly sliced
- 1-inch piece of ginger, thinly sliced

Preparation:

1. Fill a pitcher with water.
2. Add lemon and ginger slices.
3. Let infuse overnight in the refrigerator.
4. Drink throughout the next day, starting on an empty stomach in themorning.

How to Use: For at least one week, eat once a day to aid in cleaning and digesting.

Beet and Carrot Detox Juice

Intended Use: nutrient-dense beets and carrots improve blood cleansing and liver detoxification.

Ingredients:

- 2 medium beets, peeled and chopped
- 4 carrots, peeled and chopped
- ½ lemon, peeled
- 1-inch piece of fresh ginger

Preparation:

1. Juice all ingredients in a juicer.
2. Stir the juice to combine.
3. Drink immediately for maximum nutrient absorption.

How to Use: Drink one glass every day, ideally first thing in the morning, to assist the body's natural detoxifying processes.

Cilantro Heavy Metal Cleansing Pesto

Intended Use: uses the detoxifying qualities of cilantro to help the body eliminate heavy metals.

Ingredients:

- 2 cups fresh cilantro leaves
- ½ cup almonds or walnuts
- 2 garlic cloves
- ½ cup olive oil
- Juice of 1 lemon
- Salt to taste

Preparation:

1. Blend cilantro, nuts, garlic, and lemon juice in a food processor.
2. Gradually add olive oil until a smooth paste forms.
3. Season with salt.

How to Use: To help with heavy metal detoxification, use this pesto in meals on a regular basis. Examples of such meals are spaghetti and toast.

Ginger-Dandelion Detox Tea

Intended Use: benefits liver health and cleansing by using dandelion root's inherent diuretic qualities.

Ingredients:

- 1 tbsp dried dandelion root
- 1 cup boiling water

Preparation:

1. Steep dandelion root in boiling water for 10 minutes.
2. Strain and serve the tea.
3. Drink warm or at room temperature.

How to Use: Have one or two glasses daily; this helps stimulate digestion greatly in the morning.

Green Juice Detox

Intended Use: Provides a chlorophyll-rich drink to support detoxificationand boost energy levels.

Ingredients:

- 1 cup spinach
- 1 cup kale
- 1 green apple, cored and sliced
- ½ cucumber
- 1 tbsp chia seeds
- 1 cup coconut water

Preparation:

1. Combine all ingredients in a blender.
2. Blend until smooth.
3. Drink immediately.

How to Use: Enjoy this smoothie as a morning or midday drink to supportdaily detoxification and energy.

Psyllium Husk and Apple Cider Vinegar Digestive Cleanse

Intended Use: uses psyllium husk and apple cider vinegar to help encourage regularity and aid in digestive system cleaning.

Ingredients:

- 2 tbsp apple cider vinegar
- 1 tsp psyllium husk powder
- 1 cup water

Preparation:

1. Mix apple cider vinegar and psyllium husk powder in water.
2. Drink quickly before the mixture thickens.
3. Follow with another glass of water.

How to Use: Take once a day for a week to help cleanse the digestive system, ideally right before bed.

Activated Charcoal Lemonade for the Removal of Toxins

Intended Use: uses activated charcoal to aid in the absorption of toxins from the digestive tract.

Ingredients:

- 1 tsp activated charcoal powder (from coconut shells)
- Juice of 1 lemon
- 1 tbsp honey
- 1 liter of water

Preparation:

1. Dissolve activated charcoal in a small amount of water to make apaste.
2. Mix the charcoal paste with lemon juice, honey, and the rest of thewater.
3. Stir well until fully combined.

How to Use: For up to three days, have one glass of this lemonade every day to help with toxin absorption and removal.

Drink with Turmeric and Cayenne Liver Flush

Intended Use: uses cayenne pepper and turmeric to boost the body's natural detoxification processes while stimulating liver function.

Ingredients:

- 1 tsp turmeric powder
- A pinch of cayenne pepper
- Juice of 1 lemon
- 1 cup warm water
- 1 tsp honey (optional)

Preparation:

1. Mix turmeric, cayenne pepper, and lemon juice in warm water.
2. Add honey if desired for taste.
3. Stir well and drink.

How to Use: For seven days, drink this beverage first thing in the morning on an empty stomach to aid with detoxifying.

Pineapple Detox Smoothie with Spirulina

Intended Use: uses pineapple bromelain and the nutrient-rich algae spirulina to support the body's detoxification processes.

Ingredients:

- 1 tsp spirulina powder
- 1 cup pineapple chunks
- 1 banana
- 1 cup spinach
- 1 cup water or almond milk

Preparation:

1. Place all ingredients in a blender.
2. Blend until smooth.
3. Serve immediately.

How to Use: Once a day, preferably in the morning, have this smoothie to aid in the body's cleansing and nutritional absorption.

Cucumber and Aloe Vera Hydration Drink

Intended Use: hydrates and aids in detoxifying thanks to the calming effects of cucumber and aloe vera.

Ingredients:

- 2 tbsp aloe vera gel (freshly extracted or store-bought)
- ½ cucumber, blended
- Juice of ½ lemon
- 1 liter of water

Preparation:

1. Mix aloe vera gel, cucumber puree, and lemon juice in water.
2. Stir well to ensure the aloe vera is fully dissolved.
3. Refrigerate for at least an hour before serving.

How to Use: Consume throughout the day to stay hydrated and support thebody's natural detoxification processes.

HERBAL SOLUTIONS FOR KIDS

Ginger Honey Cough Syrup

Intended Use: relieves children's sore throats and coughs.

Ingredients:

- 1 cup fresh ginger, chopped
- 2 cups water
- ½ cup honey (only for children over 1 year old)

Preparation:

1. Combine ginger and water in a pot and bring to a boil. Simmer for 20minutes.
2. Strain the ginger pieces from the liquid and let it cool.
3. Stir in honey until well combined.
4. Store in a glass jar in the refrigerator.

How to Use: When your child starts to cough, give them 1 tsp of syrup. Children under the age of one should not be given honey since it might cause botulism.

Sleep Aid with Lavender Oil

Intended Use: Calms and relaxes children to promote better sleep.

Ingredients:

- 1 tbsp carrier oil (such as coconut or almond oil)
- 2 drops lavender essential oil

Preparation:

1. Mix the lavender oil with the carrier oil thoroughly.
2. Store in a small bottle.

How to Use: When your child starts to cough, give them 1 tsp of syrup. Children under the age of one should not be given honey since it might cause botulism.

Tea with Chamomile, Calming for Sleep

Intended Use: Helps children relax and promotes a peaceful sleep.

Ingredients:

- 1 tsp dried chamomile flowers
- 1 cup boiling water
- Honey (optional, for children over 1 year old)

Preparation:

1. Place chamomile flowers in a tea infuser or teapot.
2. Pour boiling water over chamomile and steep for 5 minutes.
3. Remove chamomile and let the tea cool to a suitable temperature forchildren.
4. Add a small amount of honey for sweetness if desired and approvedfor the child's age.

How to Use: To assist your youngster in relaxing and getting ready for bed, provide this tea half an hour before bed. Make sure it's cold enough to consume without risk.

Calendula External Gel

Intended Use: soothes small wounds, scrapes, and skin irritations.

Ingredients:

- ¼ cup dried calendula flowers
- ½ cup carrier oil (olive or almond oil)

Preparation:

1. Combine calendula flowers and carrier oil in a jar.
2. Seal the jar and place it in a warm, sunny spot for 2 weeks to infuse.
3. Strain out the flowers and store the oil in a clean jar.

How to Use: Two to three times a day, apply a tiny quantity to the afflicted region until the irritation subsides. Apply not to open wounds.

Tea with Peppermint for Digestion

Intended Use: reduces stomach discomfort and enhances digestion.

Ingredients:

- 1 tsp dried peppermint leaves
- 1 cup boiling water

Preparation:

1. Steep peppermint leaves in boiling water for 10 minutes.
2. Strain and let the tea cool to a child-friendly temperature.

How to Use: Give your child some to drink to help with digestion after meals or when they have a stomach pain. Make sure it's cold enough to consume without risk.

Oatmeal Bath for Itchy Skin

Intended Use: soothes itchy skin , rashes or chickenpox pain.

Ingredients:

- 1 cup finely ground oatmeal (colloidal oatmeal)
- Warm bath water

Preparation:

1. Add the colloidal oatmeal to a warm bath.
2. Stir until the oatmeal is well dispersed in the water.

How to Use: Have your child soak in the oatmeal bath for 15-20 minutes tosoothe itchy skin. No need to rinse off after the bath.

Elderberry Syrup to Boost Immunity

Intended Use: Supports the immune system to help prevent colds and flu.

Ingredients:

- ½ cup dried elderberries
- 3 cups water
- 1 cup honey (for children over 1 year old)

Preparation:

1. Combine elderberries and water in a pot; bring to a boil, then simmerfor 45 minutes.
2. Mash the berries, then strain the mixture to remove solids.
3. Let the liquid cool, then mix in the honey.
4. Store in a glass bottle in the refrigerator.

How to Use: To strengthen immunity throughout the cold and flu season, give your child 1 tsp daily. If they begin to exhibit cold symptoms, up the dosage to three times per day.

Gel of Aloe Vera for Sunburn

Intended Use: Soothes and heals sunburned skin.

Ingredients:

- Fresh aloe vera leaf or 100% pure aloe vera gel

Preparation:

1. If using a fresh leaf, slice it open and extract the gel.
2. Apply the gel directly to the sunburned area.

How to Use: Until the skin recovers, apply aloe vera gel to the burnt region two to three times a day. Any extra gel from a fresh leaf should be refrigerated.

Tea with Nettle Leaf for Allergies

Intended Use: Helps to alleviate allergy symptoms.

Ingredients:

- 1 tsp dried nettle leaves
- 1 cup boiling water

Preparation:

1. Steep nettle leaves in boiling water for 10 minutes.
2. Strain and let the tea cool to a suitable temperature.

How to Use: During allergy season, give your child up to two glasses of this tea each day to help alleviate symptoms. Make sure it's cold enough to consume without risk.

Carrot and Apple Juice for Eye Health

Intended Use: uses the vitamins and minerals in carrots and apples to support eye health and vision.

Ingredients:

- 2 carrots, washed and cut into chunks
- 1 apple, cored and sliced
- Water (optional, for blending)

Preparation:

1. Juice the carrots and apple in a juicer.
2. If using a blender, blend carrots and apple with a little water, thenstrain.

How to Use: Serve your child this juice a few times a week to support theireye health.

IMPROVED BLOOD CIRCULATION

Tea with Ginger and Cayenne Warming

Intended Use: This tea combines the warming effects of ginger with the circulatory advantages of cayenne to promote blood circulation and warmth.

Ingredients:

- 1 inch of fresh ginger root, thinly sliced
- A pinch of cayenne pepper
- 2 cups of water
- 1 tsp of honey (optional)
- Lemon slice (optional)

Preparation:

1. Bring water to a boil in a small pot.
2. Add ginger slices and simmer for 10 minutes.
3. Remove from heat and stir in a pinch of cayenne pepper.
4. Strain the tea into a mug.
5. Sweeten with honey and add a slice of lemon if desired.

How to Use: When you feel chilly, or even in the morning, have a cup of this tea to help stimulate your circulation. Start with a little dosage of cayenne and increase or decrease based on your tolerance.

Thyme and Rosemary Foot Soak

Intended Use: A foot soak that is particularly helpful for people with cold feet or poor circulation, as it combines the stimulating qualities of rosemary and thyme to enhance circulation in the extremities.

Ingredients:

- ¼ cup of dried rosemary
- ¼ cup of dried thyme
- 4 cups of hot water

Preparation:

1. Place rosemary and thyme in a large basin.
2. Pour hot water over the herbs and let steep for 10 minutes.
3. Once the water is at a comfortable temperature, soak your feet for20-30 minutes.

How to Use: As part of your nightly ritual, especially in the winter or after extended hours of sitting, use this soak.

Walnut and Pumpkin Seed Snack Mix

Intended Use: A nutrient-dense snack mix that is high in magnesium and omega-3 fatty acids from walnuts and pumpkin seeds, which are proven to promote heart health and blood flow.

Ingredients:

- ½ cup of walnuts
- ½ cup of pumpkin seeds
- A pinch of Himalayan pink salt
- A drizzle of olive oil

Preparation:

1. Preheat your oven to 160°C (320°F).
2. In a bowl, toss walnuts and pumpkin seeds with olive oil andHimalayan pink salt.
3. Spread the mix on a baking sheet and bake for 10 minutes, stirringhalfway through.
4. Let cool before serving.

How to Use: Every day, take a handful of this snack mix as a mid-morning snack or anytime you need a pick-me-up.

Smoothie with Beetroot and Orange Circulation

Intended Use: Utilizing the vitamin C from oranges and the nitrate content of beetroot, this smoothie supports cardiovascular health and improves blood flow.

Ingredients:

- 1 medium beetroot, peeled and chopped
- 1 orange, peeled and deseeded
- ½ cup of fresh strawberries

- 1 tbsp of flaxseeds
- 1 cup of water or coconut water

Preparation:

1. Place all ingredients in a blender.
2. Blend on high until smooth.
3. If the smoothie is too thick, add a bit more water or coconut water toachieve desired consistency.

How to Use: To be energized and to encourage blood circulation throughout the day, have this smoothie in the morning.

Herbal Tincture with Hawthorn Berries

Intended Use: The hawthorn fruit is well known for its heart-healthy properties, which include lowering blood pressure and increasing blood flow. A concentrated version of this tincture is used to assist cardiovascular health.

Ingredients:

- ½ cup of dried hawthorn berries
- 1 cup of vodka or apple cider vinegar (for a non-alcoholic version)
- A glass jar with a tight-fitting lid

Preparation:

1. Place hawthorn berries in the glass jar.
2. Pour vodka or apple cider vinegar over the berries, ensuring they arecompletely covered.
3. Seal the jar and store in a cool, dark place for 4 weeks, shaking itevery few days.
4. After 4 weeks, strain the tincture through a fine mesh strainer orcheesecloth into a clean bottle.

How to Use: Three times a day, take 20–30 drops of the tincture with a small amount of water. When determining tolerance, always start with a smaller dosage.

Garlic and Lemon Circulation Dressing

Intended Use: A tasty dressing that improves vascular health and blood circulation by combining the blood-thinning effects of garlic with the vitamin C content of lemon.

Ingredients:

- 2 cloves of garlic, finely minced
- Juice of 1 lemon
- ½ cup of extra virgin olive oil
- Salt and pepper to taste

Preparation:

1. In a small bowl, whisk together the lemon juice and minced garlic.
2. Slowly drizzle in the olive oil while whisking to emulsify.
3. Season with salt and pepper.
4. Store in an airtight container in the refrigerator.

How to Use: Make sure to include these items that promote circulation in your diet on a regular basis by using this dressing on cooked vegetables or salads.

Enhancing Circulation with Herbal Bath

Intended Use: a soothing bath that encourages blood flow and lowers stress by utilizing the circulatory advantages of aromatic oils and the warming effects of ginger.

Ingredients:

- 2 tbsp of fresh grated ginger
- 5 drops of cypress essential oil
- 5 drops of juniper berry essential oil
- A full bathtub of warm water

Preparation:

1. Fill your bathtub with warm water, ensuring it's at acomfortable temperature.
2. While the tub is filling, grate 2 tbsp of fresh ginger.
3. Once the tub is filled, add the grated ginger directly to the bathwater.
4. Add 5 drops each of cypress and juniper berry essential oils to the water. These oils are known for their ability to stimulate blood flow and enhance circulation.
5. Stir the bathwater gently with your hand to evenly distribute the ginger and essential oils.
6. Soak in the bath for 20-30 minutes, allowing the therapeutic properties of the ingredients to work. The warm water will aid in dilating blood vessels, improving circulation, while the ginger and essential oils will provide a warming sensation and

further boost blood flow.

How to Use: Take this herbal bath up to twice a week for maximum advantages, especially if you have slow circulation or chilly extremities. It's also a fantastic way to relax and release tension after a demanding day.

Trail Mix with Nuts and Seeds

Intended Use: A healthy snack rich in omega-3 fatty acids from nuts and seeds, which are believed to enhance blood flow by lowering inflammation and maintaining the integrity of blood vessels.

Ingredients:

- ¼ cup walnuts
- ¼ cup almonds
- ¼ cup pumpkin seeds
- ¼ cup sunflower seeds
- Optional: a sprinkle of dark chocolate chips for added antioxidants

Preparation:

1. Combine walnuts, almonds, pumpkin seeds, and sunflower seeds in a
2. large bowl.
3. If desired, add a sprinkle of dark chocolate chips to the mix for anextra antioxidant boost.
4. Toss the mixture until well combined.
5. Store the trail mix in an airtight container for easy snacking.

How to Use: Every day, have a tiny handful of this trail mix as a snack to help your blood flow. Nuts and seeds are a great source of magnesium and healthy lipids for heart health.

Golden Milk for Circulation

Intended Use: Golden milk is a warm, turmeric-based beverage that uses black pepper and turmeric's anti-inflammatory qualities to increase absorption and promote blood flow.

Ingredients:

- 1 cup of almond milk or coconut milk
- 1 tsp turmeric powder

- A pinch of ground black pepper
- 1 tsp honey (optional)
- ½ tsp ginger powder

Preparation:

1. Heat the almond milk or coconut milk in a small saucepan overmedium heat until warm (not boiling).
2. Stir in the turmeric and ginger powder, then add a pinch of blackpepper to enhance turmeric's absorption.
3. Remove from heat and sweeten with honey if desired.
4. Pour into a mug and enjoy warm.

How to Use: Have a cup of golden milk in the evening to unwind before going to bed or to promote blood flow and muscle healing after working out. For those with weak circulation or during the winter months, its warming effects are very helpful.

Rub with Hot Pepper and Garlic Oil

Intended Use: This topical oil rub combines the heat of hot peppers (capsaicin) with the circulation-enhancing properties of garlic to create a powerful remedy for improving blood flow and warming cold extremities.

Ingredients:

- 1 tbsp of finely ground hot pepper (cayenne or similar)
- 2 cloves of garlic, minced
- ½ cup of olive oil or almond oil

Preparation:

1. Gently warm the olive oil or almond oil in a saucepan over low heat.
2. Add the minced garlic and ground hot pepper to the oil, and simmer gently for 2-3 minutes. Be careful not to overheat and burn theingredients.
3. Remove from heat and let the mixture cool to room temperature.
4. Strain the oil through a fine mesh strainer or cheesecloth into a clean bottle, removing the solid particles.
5. Store the infused oil in a dark, cool place.

How to Use: Take this herbal bath up to twice a week to get the most out of it, especially if you have chilly extremities or poor circulation. After a demanding day, it's a fantastic way to relax and release tension.

BLOOD SUGAR REGULATION

Bitter Stir-Fry with Melon

Intended Use: Because of its ability to function similarly to insulin, bitter melon is a useful natural treatment for controlling blood sugar levels and promoting the health of diabetics.

Ingredients:

- 1 bitter melon
- 1 tbsp olive oil
- 2 cloves garlic, minced
- Salt to taste
- 1 onion, sliced
- 1 bell pepper, sliced

Preparation:

1. Cut the bitter melon in half, scoop out the seeds, and slice thinly.
2. Heat olive oil in a pan over medium heat.
3. Sauté garlic, onion, and bell pepper until fragrant.
4. Add the bitter melon slices and stir-fry for 5-7 minutes.
5. Season with salt according to taste.

How to Use: Include this stir-fry in your meals two or three times a week. The best results from bitter melon come from frequent consumption as part of a healthy diet.

Herbal Tea for Diabetes

Intended Use: A herbal tea mix that combines the effects of blueberry leaves, which have been demonstrated to assist control blood glucose levels, and gymnema sylvestre, dubbed the "sugar destroyer," to improve blood sugar regulation.

Ingredients:

- 1 tsp dried gymnema sylvestre leaves
- 1 tsp dried blueberry leaves
- 2 cups boiling water

Preparation:

1. Place both herbs in a teapot or a large mug.
2. Pour boiling water over the herbs and cover.
3. Let steep for 10 minutes.
4. Strain and serve.

How to Use: Have one cup of this tea every day, ideally first thing in the morning, to help control blood sugar levels. Maintaining consistency is essential to reaping the benefits.

Water with Cinnamon Fenugreek

Intended Use: This easy recipe uses fenugreek to slow down the stomach's absorption of sugar and cinnamon to increase insulin sensitivity in an effort to control blood sugar levels.

Ingredients:

- 1 tsp of ground cinnamon
- 1 tsp of fenugreek seeds
- 1 liter of water

Preparation:

1. Soak fenugreek seeds in a liter of water overnight.
2. The next morning, strain the seeds and add ground cinnamon to thewater.
3. Stir well to ensure the cinnamon is dispersed throughout the water.

How to Use: Thirty minutes before meals, have a glass of this infusion to help control blood sugar levels. For optimum benefits, carry out this exercise every day.

Avocado Cucumber Salad

Intended Use: Cucumber's high fiber content aids in blood sugar regulation, while avocado's abundance of monounsaturated fats might enhance insulin sensitivity. This salad is a healthy addition to any meal for those monitoring their blood sugar.

Ingredients:

- 1 ripe avocado, diced
- 1 cucumber, sliced
- Juice of 1 lemon
- Fresh dill, chopped
- Salt and pepper to taste

Preparation:

1. In a salad bowl, combine diced avocado and sliced cucumber.
2. Squeeze fresh lemon juice over the top.
3. Season with salt, pepper, and fresh dill.
4. Gently toss to combine.

How to Use: To help control blood sugar, try having this salad as a side dish with your main meals at least once a day.

Smoothie with Kale and Spinach

Intended Use: The magnesium and fiber found in spinach and kale, which are essential for blood sugar management and general metabolic health, are abundant in this green smoothie.

Ingredients:

- 1 cup fresh spinach
- 1 cup fresh kale, stems removed
- 1 green apple, cored and sliced
- ½ cucumber, sliced
- 1 tbsp ground flaxseeds
- 2 cups water or unsweetened almond milk

Preparation:

1. Combine spinach, kale, apple, cucumber, and ground flaxseeds in ablender.
2. Add water or almond milk to help blend the ingredients smoothly.
3. Blend on high until the mixture is completely smooth.
4. Taste and adjust the sweetness by adding more apple if needed.

How to Use: Enjoy this smoothie as a wholesome afternoon snack or to start your day off right in the morning. For people who want to naturally control their blood sugar levels, it is really helpful.

Ginger-Dandelion Detox Tea

Intended Use: Tea made from dandelion root promotes liver health and cleansing, both of which are essential for sustaining stable blood sugar levels.

Ingredients:

- 1 tbsp dried dandelion root
- 2 cups boiling water
- Lemon slice and honey (optional)

Preparation:

1. Add dried dandelion root to boiling water in a pot.
2. Cover and simmer for 10 minutes.
3. Strain the tea into mugs.
4. Add a slice of lemon and honey to taste if desired.

How to Use: Drink one cup of dandelion root tea every day, ideally first thing in the morning, to aid in the processes of detoxification and blood sugar management.

Oatmeal with Chia and Oats

Intended Use: Chia seeds contribute extra fiber and omega-3 fatty acids, which intensify the blood sugar-stabilizing properties of the pudding. Oats are an excellent source of soluble fiber, which can help control blood sugar levels.

Ingredients:

- ½ cup rolled oats
- 2 tbsp chia seeds
- 1 cup almond milk
- ½ tsp vanilla extract
- ½ cup mixed berries

Preparation:

1. In a bowl, mix oats, chia seeds, almond milk, and vanilla extract.
2. Cover and refrigerate overnight.
3. The next morning, stir the pudding and adjust the consistency withmore almond milk if needed.
4. Top with mixed berries before serving.

How to Use: Savor this pudding for breakfast to help maintain stable blood sugar levels throughout the day.

Morning Elixir with Lemon and Apple Cider Vinegar

Intended Use: It has been demonstrated that using apple cider vinegar after eating lowers blood sugar levels and increases insulin sensitivity. This elixir can be an effective strategy for controlling blood sugar swings when used with lemon.

Ingredients:

- 1 tbsp apple cider vinegar
- Juice of ½ lemon
- 1 cup warm water
- Honey (optional)

Preparation:

1. Mix apple cider vinegar and lemon juice in warm water.
2. Stir well until fully combined.
3. Add honey to taste if desired.

How to Use: Consume this concoction first thing in the morning on an empty stomach to assist in controlling your blood sugar levels all day. Give yourself at least thirty minutes to have breakfast.

Berry and Walnut Yogurt Parfait

Intended Use: This parfait blends the natural sweetness of berries and the texture of walnuts to produce a filling meal that helps control blood sugar levels. It is a well-balanced combination of protein, healthy fats, and antioxidants.

Ingredients:

- ½ cup plain Greek yogurt
- ¼ cup fresh mixed berries (blueberries, raspberries, strawberries)
- 2 tbsp chopped walnuts
- A drizzle of raw honey (optional)

Preparation:

1. Spoon half of the Greek yogurt into a glass or bowl.
2. Add a layer of mixed berries over the yogurt.
3. Sprinkle half of the chopped walnuts on top of the berries.
4. Repeat the layers with the remaining yogurt, berries, and walnuts.

5. Drizzle with raw honey if a sweeter taste is desired.

How to Use: Consume this parfait for breakfast or as a midday snack to help you keep your blood sugar levels steady all day.

Stir-fried Broccoli and Cauliflower

Intended Use: This stir-fry is a great way to control blood sugar because it's low in carbs and high in fiber. Broccoli and cauliflower are both high-nutrient veggies that promote healthy metabolism.

Ingredients:

- 1 cup cauliflower florets
- 1 cup broccoli florets
- 1 tbsp olive oil
- 2 cloves garlic, minced
- Soy sauce to taste
- Sesame seeds for garnish

Preparation:

1. Heat olive oil in a large skillet over medium heat.
2. Add minced garlic and sauté until fragrant.
3. Add cauliflower and broccoli florets, stirring frequently.
4. Cook until vegetables are tender but still crisp, about 5-7 minutes.
5. Season with soy sauce to taste.
6. Garnish with sesame seeds before serving.

How to Use: Incorporate this stir-fry into your meals 2-3 times a week. It's not only beneficial for blood sugar regulation but also adds valuable nutrientsto your diet.

HEART-WELLING SUPPORT

Tea with Hawthorn Berries

Intended Use: enhances cardiovascular health by lowering blood pressure, enhancing cardiac muscle strength, and increasing blood flow.

Ingredients:

- 1 tbsp dried hawthorn berries
- 1 cup boiling water
- Honey (optional)

Preparation:

1. Place dried hawthorn berries in a tea infuser or directly in a cup.
2. Pour boiling water over the berries and cover the cup.
3. Steep for 15 minutes.
4. Remove the infuser or strain the tea.
5. Sweeten with honey if desired.

How to Use: Sip one to two glasses per day to promote heart health. Tea made from hawthorn berries is particularly advantageous for people who have a family history of cardiovascular disease.

Dressing with Garlic and Olive Oil

Intended Use: Garlic is well recognized for its potential to reduce cholesterol and blood pressure, while olive oil's high monounsaturated fat content is good for heart health.

Ingredients:

- ½ cup extra virgin olive oil
- 3 cloves garlic, minced
- 2 tbsp apple cider vinegar
- 1 tsp Dijon mustard
- Salt and pepper to taste

Preparation:

1. In a small bowl, whisk together olive oil, minced garlic, apple cidervinegar, and

Dijon mustard.
2. Season with salt and pepper according to taste.
3. Store in an airtight container in the refrigerator.

How to Use: Include heart-healthy garlic and olive oil into your diet on a daily basis by using this dressing as a marinade or on salads.

Carrot and Beet Juice

Intended Use: Rich in nitrates and antioxidants, beets and carrots boost cardiovascular health by enhancing blood flow and lowering blood pressure.

Ingredients:

- 2 medium beets, peeled and chopped
- 4 large carrots, peeled and chopped
- 1 inch ginger root, peeled
- ½ lemon, peeled

Preparation:

1. Pass beets, carrots, ginger, and lemon through a juicer.
2. Stir the juice to combine.
3. Serve immediately or store in the refrigerator for up to 24 hours.

How to Use: To get the most out of this juice's cardiovascular advantages, have a glass in the morning on an empty stomach.

Rich in Omega-3 Flaxseed Crackers

Intended Use: High in omega-3 fatty acids, these crackers can help reduceinflammation and support heart health.

Ingredients:

- 1 cup ground flaxseeds
- ½ cup water
- 1 tsp garlic powder
- 1 tsp onion powder
- Sea salt to taste

Preparation:

1. Preheat oven to 350°F (175°C).
2. Mix ground flaxseeds with water and let sit for 5 minutes until itforms a gel-like consistency.
3. Add garlic powder, onion powder, and sea salt to the flaxseedmixture and mix well.
4. Spread the mixture thinly over a baking sheet lined with parchmentpaper.
5. Bake for 20-25 minutes or until crispy.
6. Let cool and break into cracker-sized pieces.

How to Use: Eat these crackers as a meal or as a snack to increase your consumption of heart-healthy omega-3 fatty acids.

Walnut and spinach salad

Intended Use: Walnuts contain omega-3 fatty acids, while spinach is rich in potassium and magnesium, all of which are vital for heart health. The abundance of nutrients in this salad promotes cardiovascular health.

Ingredients:

- 2 cups fresh spinach leaves
- ½ cup walnuts, chopped
- ¼ cup dried cranberries
- Dressing: 3 tbsp balsamic vinegar, 1 tbsp olive oil, salt,and pepper

Preparation:

1. In a large bowl, combine spinach leaves, chopped walnuts, and driedcranberries.
2. In a small bowl, whisk together balsamic vinegar, olive oil, salt, andpepper to make the dressing.
3. Drizzle the dressing over the salad and toss gently to combine.

How to Use: To get the benefits of its heart-healthy elements, serve this salad as a side dish with your meals at least three times a week.

Turmeric Ginger Heart Tonic

Intended Use: Due to its anti-inflammatory qualities, ginger and turmeric can both lower cardiovascular risk factors.

Ingredients:

- 1 tsp turmeric powder

- 1 tsp ginger powder
- 2 cups water
- Honey and lemon juice to taste

Preparation:

1. Add turmeric and ginger powder to boiling water.
2. Reduce heat and simmer for 10 minutes.
3. Strain the tonic into a mug.
4. Add honey and lemon juice according to taste.

How to Use: Take one daily glass of this tonic, especially in the morning, to get the advantages of ginger and turmeric for your cardiovascular system.

Pudding with Chia Seeds and Berries

Intended Use: Omega-3 fatty acids are essential for heart health and are abundant in chia seeds. Antioxidants from berries can prevent heart disease.

Ingredients:

- ¼ cup chia seeds
- 1 cup almond milk
- ½ tsp vanilla extract
- 1 cup mixed berries

Preparation:

1. In a bowl, mix chia seeds with almond milk and vanilla extract.
2. Let the mixture sit for at least 30 minutes or overnight in therefrigerator until it becomes pudding-like.
3. Top with mixed berries before serving.

How to Use: Eat this pudding for breakfast or as a dessert to increase your consumption of antioxidants and heart-healthy omega-3 fatty acids.

Avocado with Cacao Smoothie

Intended Use: Avocado has heart-healthy lipids that lower cholesterol, while cacao has a high concentration of antioxidants that promote heart health.

Ingredients:

- 1 ripe avocado
- 2 tbsp raw cacao powder
- 1 banana
- 1 cup spinach
- 1 cup almond milk
- Ice cubes (optional)

Preparation:

1. Combine all ingredients in a blender.
2. Blend until smooth.
3. Add ice cubes for a colder smoothie if desired.

How to Use: To get the advantages of this smoothie's cardiovascular properties, drink it frequently as a wholesome snack or as a meal replacement.

Vegetable and Lentil Stew

Intended Use: Lentils are a great source of plant-based protein and fiber, which help reduce the risk of heart disease. This stew also packs a variety of vegetables for additional nutrients and antioxidants.

Ingredients:

- 1 cup dried lentils, rinsed
- 4 cups vegetable broth
- 1 onion, diced
- 2 carrots, diced
- 2 stalks celery, diced
- 1 can diced tomatoes
- 1 tsp each of dried thyme and rosemary
- Salt and pepper to taste

Preparation:

1. In a large pot, sauté onion, carrots, and celery until softened.
2. Add lentils, vegetable broth, diced tomatoes, thyme, and rosemary.
3. Bring to a boil, then reduce heat and simmer, covered, for about 30 minutes or until lentils are tender.
4. Season with salt and pepper to taste.

How to Use: This stew may be served as a filling supper at any time of day. It's particularly helpful in the winter months when the body longs for comforting, nutrient-dense meals.

Oatmeal for Heart Health

Intended Use: Soluble fiber, which helps decrease cholesterol and enhance heart health, is abundant in oatmeal.

Ingredients:

- 1 cup rolled oats
- 2 cups water or almond milk
- 1 apple, diced
- 1 tsp cinnamon
- 1 tbsp flaxseeds

Preparation:

1. Cook oats in water or almond milk according to package instructions.
2. Stir in diced apple and cinnamon during the last few minutes ofcooking.
3. Sprinkle with flaxseeds before serving.

How to Use: Eat this heart-healthy oatmeal for breakfast to provide your body with a nutritious start to the day.

DETOXIFICATION AND SKIN CLEANING

Herbal Dandelion Tea

Intended Use: aids in kidney and liver cleansing and has diuretic qualities to aid in the removal of pollutants.

Ingredients:

- 1 tbsp dried dandelion leaves
- 1 cup boiling water

Preparation:

1. Place dried dandelion leaves in a teapot or cup.
2. Pour boiling water over the leaves and steep for 10 minutes.
3. Strain and drink warm.

How to Use: To assist the body's natural detoxification processes, drink two to three cups every day for a week.

Lemonade with Activated Charcoal

Intended Use: Utilizes the binding properties of activated charcoal to absorband help remove toxins from the digestive system.

Ingredients:

- Juice of 1 lemon
- 1 tsp activated charcoal powder
- 1 tbsp maple syrup
- 1 cup water

Preparation:

1. In a glass, combine lemon juice, activated charcoal, and maple syrup.
2. Add water and stir until well mixed.
3. Drink immediately.

How to Use: Drink this beverage once daily for three days as part of your cleansing routine. Take neither with other vitamins nor prescription drugs.

Super Detox Drink

Intended Use: supports liver function and bloodstream cleansing by offering a wealth of antioxidants, vitamins, and minerals that aid in the body's detoxification process.

Ingredients:

- 1 cup fresh spinach
- ½ cup cilantro
- 1 apple, cored and sliced
- 1 banana
- 1 tbsp chia seeds
- 1 cup coconut water
- Juice of ½ lemon

Preparation:

1. Place spinach, cilantro, apple, banana, and chia seeds into a blender.
2. Add coconut water and lemon juice.
3. Blend on high until smooth.
4. Serve immediately for maximum nutrient retention.

How to Use: Drink this smoothie once a day, ideally first thing in the morning when you're not hungry, to help your body rid itself of toxins.

Turmeric and Ginger Detox Tea

Intended Use: uses ginger's digestive help and turmeric's anti-inflammatory qualities to aid in detoxifying and relieve inflammation.

Ingredients:

- 1 inch fresh ginger root, thinly sliced
- 1 tsp turmeric powder
- 4 cups water
- Honey to taste (optional)

Preparation:

1. Add ginger slices and turmeric to water in a pot.
2. Bring to a boil, then simmer for 10-15 minutes.
3. Strain into a cup and add honey if desired.

How to Use: To assist with detoxification and to lower inflammation, have one to two cups per day.

Cucumber Mint Water for Cleaning

Intended Use: Cucumber and mint's cooling, diuretic qualities hydrate and aid in the removal of impurities from the body.

Ingredients:

- 1 cucumber, thinly sliced
- 10 mint leaves
- 2 liters of water

Preparation:

1. In a large pitcher, combine cucumber slices and mint leaves.
2. Fill the pitcher with water and stir.
3. Refrigerate for at least 2 hours to allow flavors to infuse.

How to Use: Drink continuously throughout the day to help with detoxification and hydration.

Beet Juice with Lemon for Liver Cleansing

Intended Use: Boosts blood purification and liver health with beetroot's detoxifying qualities and lemon's abundance of antioxidants.

Ingredients:

- 2 medium beetroots, peeled and chopped
- Juice of 1 lemon
- 1 apple, cored and chopped (optional for sweetness)
- 1 inch ginger root, peeled
- 1 cup water

Preparation:

1. Place all ingredients in a blender or juicer.
2. Blend or juice until smooth.
3. Strain if desired and drink fresh.

How to Use: To boost liver function and aid in the body's natural detoxifying processes, drink one glass per day, particularly in the morning.

Apple Cider Vinegar Morning Tonic

Intended Use: With apple cider vinegar's probiotics and acidic qualities, it stimulates digestive enzymes and aids in liver cleansing.

Ingredients:

- 2 tbsp apple cider vinegar (with "the mother")
- 1 cup warm water
- Juice of ½ lemon
- 1 tsp honey (optional)

Preparation:

1. In a glass, combine apple cider vinegar, warm water, and lemonjuice.
2. Stir well and add honey if desired for sweetness.

How to Use: On an empty stomach, sip this tonic first thing in the morning to help assist detoxification and stimulate your digestive system.

Detoxifying Soup with Broccoli

Intended Use: This soup, being high in fiber and antioxidants, aids in detoxing and offers vital nutrients for general well-being.

Ingredients:

- 2 heads of broccoli, chopped
- 1 onion, diced
- 2 cloves garlic, minced
- 4 cups vegetable broth
- Salt and pepper to taste
- 1 tbsp olive oil

Preparation:

1. In a large pot, heat olive oil over medium heat.
2. Add onion and garlic, sautéing until translucent.
3. Add broccoli and vegetable broth, bringing to a boil.
4. Reduce heat, cover, and simmer until broccoli is tender.

5. Blend the soup until smooth using an immersion blender or standblender.
6. Season with salt and pepper to taste.

How to Use: Have a cup of this soup every day to aid in nutritional intake and bodily cleaning, particularly during detox times.

Bath with seaweed detoxification

Intended Use: uses the seaweed's abundant mineral content to pull toxins out of the skin, encouraging rest and cleansing.

Ingredients:

- ½ cup dried seaweed (kelp or nori)
- Hot bathwater

Preparation:

1. Fill a bathtub with hot water.
2. Add dried seaweed directly to the bath or in a muslin bag to preventclogging.
3. Soak in the bath for 20-30 minutes.

How to Use: Once or twice a week, treat yourself to a seaweed detox bath to aid in skin purification and relaxation.

Salad to Support the Liver

Intended Use: a nutrient-dense salad made with liver-friendly components to promote liver function and detoxification.

Ingredients:

- 2 cups mixed greens (spinach, arugula, kale)
- ½ cup chopped parsley
- 1 beet, grated
- 1 carrot, grated
- ¼ cup walnuts, chopped
- Dressing: 2 tbsp extra virgin olive oil, 1 tbsp lemon juice,1 tsp Dijon mustard, salt, and pepper

Preparation:

1. In a large salad bowl, combine mixed greens, parsley, grated beet,and carrot.

2. In a small bowl, whisk together olive oil, lemon juice, Dijon mustard,salt, and pepper to make the dressing.
3. Drizzle the dressing over the salad and toss to coat evenly.
4. Top with chopped walnuts before serving.

How to Use: Incorporate this salad into your daily meals to support liver health and promote detoxification. Enjoy it as a main dish or a side salad to reap the detoxifying benefits.

DIGESTIVE ENZYME SUPPORT

Papaya and Pineapple Smoothie

Intended Use: increases the synthesis of digestive enzymes, such as papain from papaya and bromelain from pineapple, which promote and help in the breakdown of proteins.

Ingredients:

- 1 cup fresh pineapple, chopped
- 1 cup fresh papaya, chopped
- 1 banana
- ½ cup coconut water or water
- 1 tsp fresh ginger, grated (optional for additional digestivesupport)

Preparation:

1. Combine pineapple, papaya, banana, and coconut water in a blender.
2. Add grated ginger if using.
3. Blend on high until smooth.
4. Serve immediately for the freshest taste and most potent enzymeactivity.

How to Use: To ensure that your digestive system is ready for the best possible performance all day, drink this smoothie in the morning or before meals.

Blend of Digestive Herbal Tea

Intended Use: uses a combination of digestive-supporting herbs to help ease discomfort associated with the digestive system and improve the body's natural synthesis of enzymes.

Ingredients:

- 1 tsp dried peppermint leaves
- 1 tsp dried fennel seeds
- 1 tsp dried chamomile flowers
- 2 cups boiling water

Preparation:

1. Combine peppermint, fennel seeds, and chamomile in a teapot orheat-proof container.

2. Pour boiling water over the herbs and cover.
3. Steep for 10 minutes, then strain.
4. Serve the tea warm, or chill it for a refreshing cold drink.

How to Use: To promote digestion, have a cup of herbal tea half an hour before eating, or after to reduce pain.

Aloe Vera Digestive Aid

Intended Use: uses the natural enzymes present in aloe vera to soothe the digestive system and aid in the absorption of nutrients.

Ingredients:

- 2 tbsp of pure aloe vera gel (ensure it's edible and free fromaloin)
- 1 cup water or a mild herbal tea

Preparation:

1. In a blender, combine the aloe vera gel and water or herbal tea.
2. Blend until smooth.
3. Serve immediately.

How to Use: To help with digestion throughout the day, drink this aloe vera drink first thing in the morning on an empty stomach.

Carrots with fermented ginger

Intended Use: provides probiotics through fermentation, which can aid in boosting the synthesis of natural digestive enzymes and promoting gut health and digestion.

Ingredients:

- 4 cups grated carrots
- 1 tbsp grated ginger
- 1 tbsp sea salt
- Purified water

Preparation:

1. In a large bowl, mix grated carrots, ginger, and sea salt.
2. Pack the mixture into a clean, sterilized jar, leaving about 2 inches ofspace at the top.

3. Add enough purified water to cover the carrots completely, ensuringthey are submerged.
4. Close the jar loosely to allow gases to escape and let it sit at roomtemperature for 3-7 days.
5. Check daily to ensure carrots are submerged, adding more water ifnecessary.
6. Once fermentation is complete, tighten the lid and store in therefrigerator.

How to Use: Every day, add a tiny quantity of fermented ginger carrots to your meals to promote gut health and facilitate digestion.

Kombucha

Intended Use: replenishes the gut with healthy microbes that help improve the body's natural synthesis of digestive enzymes.

Ingredients:

- 1 SCOBY (Symbiotic Culture Of Bacteria and Yeast)
- 8 cups of water
- 4 tea bags (green or black tea)
- 1 cup of pre-made kombucha (from a previous batch or store-bought)

Preparation:

1. Boil water.
2. Steep tea bags in the sugar water for 5-10 minutes, then remove.
3. Allow the tea to cool to room temperature, then add the SCOBY andpre-made kombucha.
4. Cover the container with a breathable cloth and secure with a rubberband.
5. Let the mixture ferment at room temperature, out of direct sunlight,for 7-14 days.
6. Taste the kombucha to determine if it has reached your desired level of fermentation.
7. Once ready, remove the SCOBY (save for the next batch) and bottlethe kombucha.

How to Use: Consume 4–8 ounces of kombucha per day to aid with digestion. Reduce the quantity at first and observe how your body responds.

Apple cider vinegar tonic for digestion

Intended Use: enhances digestion by balancing stomach acid levels and stimulating digestive enzymes.

Ingredients:

- 1 tbsp organic apple cider vinegar (with "the mother")
- 1 cup warm water
- 1 tsp honey (optional)

Preparation:

1. Mix apple cider vinegar and warm water.
2. Add honey to taste, if desired.
3. Stir well to combine.

How to Use: Use this tonic to increase the activity of digestive enzymes 20 to 30 minutes before meals.

Soup Miso with Seaweed

Intended Use: provides nutrients from seaweed and probiotics from miso, both of which enhance the formation of enzymes and the health of the digestive system.

Ingredients:

- 4 cups water
- 2 tbsp miso paste
- 1 cup chopped seaweed (nori, wakame, or kombu)
- ½ cup tofu, cubed
- Green onion for garnish

Preparation:

1. Bring water to a simmer in a pot.
2. Add seaweed and tofu, simmering for 5 minutes.
3. Remove from heat. In a separate bowl, dissolve miso paste in a smallamount of the hot broth, then add back to the pot.
4. Garnish with green onion.

How to Use: Every day, especially before or after meals, have a cup of miso soup to improve intestinal health.

Water from Chia Seeds

Intended Use: supplies fiber and water, both of which can improve the action of enzymes and assist the digestive system.

Ingredients:

- 1 tbsp chia seeds
- 1 cup water
- Juice of ½ lemon (optional)

Preparation:

1. Soak chia seeds in water for 20 minutes, allowing them to gel.
2. Add lemon juice for flavor and additional digestive support.
3. Stir well before drinking.

How to Use: Drink chia seed water first thing in the morning to help with digestion and daily hydration.

Raw Papaya Salad

Intended Use: uses papain, a natural digestive enzyme found in papayas that helps break down protein and may help minimize bloating.

Ingredients:

- 2 cups fresh papaya, thinly sliced
- Juice of 1 lime
- 1 tbsp honey
- A pinch of salt
- Fresh mint leaves for garnish

Preparation:

1. In a bowl, combine papaya slices with lime juice, honey, and salt.
2. Toss gently to coat.
3. Garnish with mint leaves before serving.

How to Use: Consume this salad as a starter or side dish to aid digestion,particularly during meals heavy in protein.

Berries and Probiotic Yogurt Parfait

Intended Use: Supports gut health with probiotics from yogurt, enhancingthe body's ability to produce digestive enzymes.

Ingredients:

- 1 cup plain probiotic yogurt
- ½ cup mixed berries (blueberries, strawberries, raspberries)
- 1 tbsp flaxseed, ground
- Honey or maple syrup to taste

Preparation:

1. Layer yogurt and berries in a glass or bowl.
2. Sprinkle ground flaxseed on top.
3. Drizzle with honey or maple syrup to taste.

How to Use: Savor this parfait for breakfast or as a snack to help your digestive system stay healthy all day. It contains probiotics.

DIGESTIVE HEALTH

Digestive Tea with Peppermint and Fennel

Intended Use: The carminative qualities of fennel and the antispasmodic qualities of peppermint help to ease stomach pain and facilitate digestion.

Ingredients:

- 1 tsp dried fennel seeds
- 1 tsp dried peppermint leaves
- 1 cup boiling water

Preparation:

1. Place fennel seeds and peppermint leaves in a tea infuser or directlyin a cup.
2. Pour boiling water over the herbs and cover.
3. Steep for 10 minutes, then strain.
4. Drink warm.

How to Use: Drink a cup of this tea to help with digestion after meals or whenever you feel uncomfortable in your stomach.

Probiotic Bowl of Yogurt

Intended Use: Yogurt's active probiotics help to improve gut flora and enhance digestive health in general.

Ingredients:

- 1 cup organic plain yogurt (ensure it contains live cultures)
- ½ cup fresh berries
- 1 tbsp ground flaxseed
- 1 tbsp honey (optional)

Preparation:

1. Spoon yogurt into a bowl.
2. Top with fresh berries and sprinkle with ground flaxseed.
3. Drizzle with honey for added sweetness if desired.

How to Use: Include in your regular breakfast regimen to promote digestion and intestinal health.

Digestive Bone Broth

Intended Use: Supports gut health and heals the digestive tract with its highcollagen content, which can help repair intestinal lining.

Ingredients:

- 2 pounds of mixed bones (chicken, beef, or fish)
- 2 carrots, chopped
- 2 celery stalks, chopped
- 1 onion, chopped
- 2 tbsp apple cider vinegar
- Herbs such as thyme and rosemary
- Water to cover

Preparation:

1. Place bones in a large pot and cover with water. Add apple cidervinegar to help leach minerals from the bones.
2. Add chopped vegetables and herbs.
3. Bring to a boil, then reduce heat and simmer for 12-24 hours. Skimoff any foam or impurities that rise to the top.
4. Strain the broth through a fine-mesh sieve and store in therefrigerator or freezer.

How to Use: To maintain digestive health, drink one cup of bone broth every day, either on its own or as a foundation for soups and stews.

Warm Lemon Water

Intended Use: helps remove toxins from the digestive tract and stimulates the enzymes involved in digestion.

Ingredients:

- Juice of ½ lemon
- 1 cup warm water

Preparation:

1. Squeeze the juice of half a lemon into a cup of warm water.
2. Stir to mix and drink warm.

How to Use: On an empty stomach, have your morning beverage to help your digestive system get going.

Apple Cider Vinegar Salad Dressing

Intended Use: Improves digestion and increases stomach acid with theprobiotic and acidic properties of apple cider vinegar.

Ingredients:

- ¼ cup apple cider vinegar (with "the mother")
- ¾ cup extra virgin olive oil
- 1 tsp mustard
- 1 tsp honey
- Salt and pepper to taste

Preparation:

1. In a jar, combine apple cider vinegar, olive oil, mustard, and honey.
2. Seal the jar and shake vigorously until well combined.
3. Season with salt and pepper to taste.

How to Use: Use this combination to dress salads and add digestive assistance to everyday meals.

Soothing Aloe Vera Drink

Intended Use: Soothes the digestive tract and aids in healing with the anti-inflammatory properties of aloe vera.

Ingredients:

- 2 tbsp of edible aloe vera gel
- 1 cup water or coconut water
- Juice of ½ lime

Preparation:

1. Blend aloe vera gel with water or coconut water until smooth.
2. Add lime juice and blend again.

3. Serve chilled for a refreshing digestive aid.

How to Use: Drink once daily, preferably in the morning, to support digestive health and soothe irritation.

Ginger Zinger Digestive Shot

Intended Use: Boosts digestion and relieves nausea with the potent anti-inflammatory properties of ginger.

Ingredients:

- 1 inch fresh ginger root
- Juice of 1 lemon
- ½ tsp cayenne pepper
- 1 tsp honey (optional)
- ¼ cup water

Preparation:

1. Blend ginger root with water until smooth.
2. Strain the mixture to extract ginger juice.
3. Mix ginger juice with lemon juice, cayenne pepper, and honey ifusing.
4. Drink immediately.

How to Use: Take this shot either before meals or in the morning to improve your digestion.

Kefir Smoothie

Intended Use: Provides a rich source of probiotics to support healthy gutflora and digestion.

Ingredients:

- 1 cup kefir
- ½ banana
- ½ cup mixed berries
- 1 tbsp chia seeds

Preparation:

1. Combine kefir, banana, berries, and chia seeds in a blender.
2. Blend until smooth.

3. Serve immediately for best taste and nutritional value.

How to Use: To enhance your probiotic consumption, have this smoothie for morning or as a snack.

Dandelion Root Digestive Bitters

Intended Use: Stimulates bile production and supports liver function withdandelion root, enhancing digestion.

Ingredients:

- 2 tbsp dried dandelion root
- 1 cup vodka or apple cider vinegar (for a non-alcoholic version)
- 1 tsp orange peel
- 1 tsp ginger root

Preparation:

1. Combine dandelion root, orange peel, and ginger root in a jar.
2. Cover with vodka or apple cider vinegar.
3. Seal the jar and let it sit in a cool, dark place for 2-4 weeks, shakingoccasionally.
4. Strain the mixture and store in a clean bottle.

How to Use: To aid with digestion, take one or two tbsp before meals.

Prebiotic Fiber-Rich Oatmeal

Intended Use: Supports gut health with a high-fiber meal that feedsbeneficial gut bacteria, enhancing digestive health.

Ingredients:

- 1 cup rolled oats
- 2 cups water or almond milk
- 1 tbsp ground flaxseeds
- ½ apple, diced
- Cinnamon to taste

Preparation:

1. Cook oats in water or almond milk according to package instructions.
2. Stir in ground flaxseeds and diced apple during the last few minutesof cooking.

3. Sprinkle with cinnamon before serving.

How to Use: For everyday digestive health support and to keep a balanced and healthy gut flora, have this high-fiber oatmeal for breakfast.

A STAMINA AND ENERGY BOOST

Maca Root Energy Smoothie

Intended Use: uses maca root, a natural adaptogen that balances hormones and improves endurance, to increase energy and stamina.

Ingredients:

- 1 tbsp maca powder
- 1 banana
- 1 cup spinach
- 1 tbsp almond butter
- 1 cup almond milk
- A handful of ice cubes

Preparation:

1. Place all ingredients in a blender.
2. Blend on high until smooth and creamy.
3. Serve immediately for the best flavor and nutrient retention.

How to Use: Drink this smoothie in the morning or right before working out to boost your energy and stamina naturally.

Beet juice with berries and beets

Intended Use: enhances blood circulation and endurance with beets and berries high in antioxidants.

Ingredients:

- 2 medium beetroots, peeled and chopped
- 1 cup mixed berries (such as strawberries, raspberries, and blueberries)
- 1 apple, cored and sliced
- ½ inch ginger, peeled

Preparation:

1. Process all ingredients through a juicer.

2. Stir the juice well to combine.
3. Serve immediately to ensure maximum nutrient intake.

How to Use: To improve your physical performance and endurance, drink this juice in the morning or before engaging in any physical activity.

Energy Bars with Chia Seeds

Intended Use: uses omega-3-rich chia seeds to deliver crucial nutrients and long-lasting energy.

Ingredients:

- 1 cup dates, pitted
- ¼ cup chia seeds
- ¼ cup flaxseeds
- ½ cup oats
- ¼ cup almond butter
- 2 tbsp honey

Preparation:

1. In a food processor, blend dates until they form a sticky paste.
2. Add chia seeds, flaxseeds, oats, almond butter, and honey to the datepaste. Pulse until well combined.
3. Press the mixture into a lined baking tray, creating a flat, even layer.
4. Refrigerate for at least 2 hours, then cut into bars.

How to Use: For an energy boost, eat one bar as needed, especially in the middle of the morning or mid-afternoon when energy tends to decline.

Herbal Tea with Ginseng

Intended Use: Increases energy levels both mentally and physically using ginseng, which is well known for its energy-enhancing qualities.

Ingredients:

- 1 tsp dried ginseng root
- 1 cup boiling water
- Honey or lemon to taste (optional)

Preparation:

1. Place ginseng root in a tea infuser or directly in a cup.
2. Pour boiling water over the ginseng and let steep for 5-10 minutes.
3. Remove the ginseng root or infuser.
4. Add honey or lemon to taste if desired.

How to Use: To increase energy levels without affecting your ability to sleep at night, have one cup of ginseng tea in the morning or early afternoon.

Energy Drink with Citrus and Spirulina

Intended Use: boosts vigor and energy with vitamin C-rich citrus fruits and nutrient-dense spirulina.

Ingredients:

- 1 tsp spirulina powder
- Juice of 1 orange
- Juice of ½ lemon
- 1 tsp honey
- 1 cup water

Preparation:

1. In a glass, combine spirulina powder with a little water to form apaste.
2. Add orange juice, lemon juice, honey, and the remaining water. Mixwell until the spirulina is fully dissolved.
3. Serve chilled or at room temperature.

How to Use: Have this energizing drink first thing in the morning to get your day going, or before you work out.

Ashwagandha and Cacao Warm Milk

Intended Use: uses antioxidant-rich cocoa and adaptogenic ashwagandha to lower stress and increase energy.

Ingredients:

- 1 tsp ashwagandha powder
- 1 tbsp raw cacao powder

- 1 cup almond milk
- Honey to taste

Preparation:

1. Heat almond milk in a small saucepan over low heat until warm.
2. Whisk in ashwagandha and cacao powder until well combined.
3. Remove from heat and sweeten with honey as desired.
4. Serve warm.

How to Use: Drink in the evening to decompress and rejuvenate, encouraging sound sleep and increased vitality the following day.

Mint and Green Tea Refresher

Intended Use: Refreshing mint and antioxidant-rich green tea boost energy and speed your metabolism.

Ingredients:

- 1 green tea bag
- 5-6 fresh mint leaves
- 1 cup boiling water
- Ice cubes (for serving cold)
- Honey to taste (optional)

Preparation:

1. Steep the green tea bag and mint leaves in boiling water for 3-5minutes.
2. Remove the tea bag and mint leaves.
3. Add honey if desired and stir until dissolved.
4. Serve hot, or chill with ice cubes for a refreshing cold drink.

How to Use: For a natural energy boost, sip on a cup of this energizing beverage in the morning or early afternoon.

Almond and Quinoa Energy Bowl

Intended Use: Offers a high-protein, nutrient-rich meal to support energylevels throughout the day.

Ingredients:

- 1 cup cooked quinoa
- ¼ cup sliced almonds
- ½ cup blueberries
- 1 tbsp chia seeds
- Honey or maple syrup to taste
- Almond milk, as desired

Preparation:

1. In a bowl, combine cooked quinoa, sliced almonds, blueberries, andchia seeds.
2. Drizzle with honey or maple syrup for sweetness.
3. Add almond milk to achieve your desired consistency.

How to Use: Savor this energy bowl for breakfast or as a filling snack to keep your energy and endurance high.

Avocado and Walnut Salad

Intended Use: provide vital nutrients and good fats for long-term energy and mental wellness.

Ingredients:

- 2 cups mixed greens (spinach, arugula, kale)
- 1 ripe avocado, diced
- ½ cup walnuts, chopped
- ¼ cup dried cranberries
- Dressing: Olive oil, lemon juice, salt, and pepper

Preparation:

1. In a large salad bowl, combine mixed greens, diced avocado,chopped walnuts, and dried cranberries.
2. In a small bowl, whisk together olive oil, lemon juice, salt, andpepper to create the dressing.
3. Drizzle the dressing over the salad and toss gently to combine.

How to Use: Consume this salad for lunch or dinner to fuel your body withhigh-quality nutrients for energy and stamina.

Electrolyte Boost with Berries and Coconut Water

Intended Use: Natural coconut water and antioxidant-rich berries hydrate and replace electrolytes, improving energy and healing.

Ingredients:

- 1 cup coconut water
- ½ cup mixed berries (fresh or frozen)
- Juice of ½ lime
- A few mint leaves for garnish

Preparation:

1. Blend coconut water, mixed berries, and lime juice until smooth.
2. Serve garnished with mint leaves.
3. Enjoy chilled for a refreshing energy boost.

How to Use: Drink to rapidly replace lost fluids and electrolytes after exercise or in hot temperatures, which will promote stamina and energy recovery.

EXTRA-INTESTINAL SOFTNESS

Aloe Vera and Honey Rejuvenating Cocktail

Intended Use: helps heal the lining of the gastrointestinal tract and calms troubled stomachs.

Ingredients:

- 2 tbsp of pure aloe vera gel (ensure it's edible)
- 1 tbsp honey
- 1 cup water

Preparation:

1. Mix aloe vera gel and honey in a glass of water until fully dissolved.
2. Stir well to ensure a uniform mixture.

How to Use: For the health and comfort of your gastrointestinal tract, take one serving each day on an empty stomach.

Fennel Seed Aid for Digestion

Intended Use: Relieves gas, bloating, and cramps associated with digestiveissues.

Ingredients:

- 1 tsp fennel seeds
- 1 cup boiling water

Preparation:

1. Crush the fennel seeds slightly to release their oil.
2. Place the crushed seeds in a cup and pour boiling water over them.
3. Cover and let steep for 10 minutes.
4. Strain and drink warm.

How to Use: After meals, sip on a cup of fennel seed tea to aid with digestion and avoid pain.

Ginger and Peppermint Digestive Tea

Intended Use: relieves stomach pain, lessens bloating, and eases digestive discomfort.

Ingredients:

- 1 tsp dried peppermint leaves
- 1 tsp grated fresh ginger
- 1 cup boiling water

Preparation:

1. Place peppermint leaves and grated ginger in a tea infuser or directlyinto a cup.
2. Pour boiling water over the leaves and ginger.
3. Cover and let steep for 10 minutes.
4. Strain (if needed) and serve warm.

How to Use: Especially after meals, drink this tea two to three times a day to help with digestion and ease pain.

Bone Broth for Healing the Gut

Intended Use: Collagen, amino acids, and minerals are used to nourish the digestive system and promote gut healing.

Ingredients:

- 2 pounds mixed beef bones (marrow and knuckle bones)
- 2 carrots, chopped
- 2 celery stalks, chopped
- 1 onion, quartered
- 2 tbsp apple cider vinegar
- Water to cover
- Salt to taste

Preparation:

1. Place bones in a large pot and cover with cold water. Add apple cidervinegar; let sit for 30 minutes.
2. Add vegetables to the pot. Bring to a boil, then reduce to a simmer.
3. Simmer for 12-24 hours, skimming foam and impurities from thesurface.
4. Strain the broth, season with salt, and cool.

5. Store in the refrigerator for up to 5 days or freeze for longer storage.

How to Use: Drink one cup of warm bone broth every day to promote comfort and good digestion.

Rich in Probiotics Sauerkraut

Intended Use: uses natural probiotics to assist overall digestive health and improve the balance of intestinal flora.

Ingredients:

- 1 medium head cabbage, shredded
- 1 tbsp sea salt

Preparation:

1. Mix cabbage and salt in a large bowl. Massage until cabbage releasesits juice.
2. Pack cabbage tightly into a clean mason jar, pressing down untiljuices cover the cabbage.
3. Cover the jar with a cloth and secure with a rubber band.
4. Let the jar sit at room temperature for 3-10 days. Check daily,pressing down the cabbage if it rises above its liquid.
5. Once fermented, seal the jar and store in the refrigerator.

How to Use: Consume a tiny amount of sauerkraut each day to help keep your gut flora and digestion in good condition.

Warm Water with Lemon and Cinnamon

Intended Use: increases gastrointestinal motility and stimulates digestion enzymes.

Ingredients:

- Juice of ½ lemon
- ½ tsp cinnamon
- 1 cup warm water

Preparation:

1. Add lemon juice and cinnamon to warm water.
2. Stir well to combine.

How to Use: Drink first thing in the morning to kickstart your digestivesystem for the day.

Comfort Herbal Digestive Capsules

Intended Use: offers a combination of herbs that are well-known for promoting digestive health and relieving pain.

Ingredients:

- Dried peppermint leaf powder
- Dried ginger root powder
- Dried fennel seed powder
- Empty capsules

Preparation:

1. In a bowl, mix equal parts of peppermint, ginger, and fennelpowders.
2. Fill empty capsules with the herbal mixture using a capsule filler or asmall spoon.
3. Store the filled capsules in a cool, dry place.

How to Use: Take one or two capsules as needed to relieve upset stomach; do not take more than six capsules in a day.

Berry-Kefir Digestive Parfait

Intended Use: Combines probiotics from kefir with fiber from berries for agut health-boosting treat.

Ingredients:

- 1 cup plain kefir
- ½ cup mixed berries (blueberries, strawberries, raspberries)
- 1 tbsp chia seeds
- Honey (optional, for sweetness)

Preparation:

1. In a glass, layer kefir, berries, and chia seeds.
2. Repeat the layers until all ingredients are used.
3. Drizzle with honey if desired.

How to Use: Enjoy as a breakfast or snack to support digestive health through a combination of probiotics and fiber.

Digestive Smoothie with Papaya

Intended Use: includes papain, a papaya enzyme that aids in protein digestion, minimizing bloating and enhancing digestive health.

Ingredients:

- 1 cup fresh papaya, chopped
- ½ banana
- 1 cup coconut water
- 1 tbsp lime juice
- A handful of ice

Preparation:

1. Place papaya, banana, coconut water, lime juice, and ice in a blender.
2. Blend until smooth.
3. Serve immediately.

How to Use: Have this smoothie in the morning or right before meals to help with digestion and to soothe your stomach.

Cucumber Mint Juice for Hydration

Intended Use: hydrates the body and aids with digestive health with a cool cucumber-mint combination.

Ingredients:

- 1 large cucumber, peeled and chopped
- 10 mint leaves
- Juice of 1 lime
- 1 cup water

Preparation:

1. Blend cucumber, mint leaves, lime juice, and water until smooth.
2. Strain the juice for a smoother texture, if desired.
3. Serve chilled.

How to Use: Drink this drink all day to help your digestive system and remain hydrated, especially after working out in the heat.

OVERALL HEALTH AND LIFESPAN

Superfood Green Juice

Intended Use: increases lifespan and general well-being with a combination of superfoods high in antioxidants.

Ingredients:

- 1 cup spinach
- 1 cup kale
- ½ avocado
- ½ cup blueberries
- 1 tbsp chia seeds
- 1 tbsp flaxseeds
- 1 tsp spirulina powder
- 2 cups water or almond milk

Preparation:

1. Wash spinach and kale thoroughly.
2. Place all ingredients in a high-powered blender.
3. Blend on high until smooth and creamy.
4. Serve immediately for the best nutritional value.

How to Use: Drink one smoothie a day, ideally in the morning, to provide essential nutrients that promote lifespan and overall well-being.

Berry and Walnut Antioxidant Salad

Intended Use: offers a nutrient-dense supper with antioxidants to improve heart health and lifespan.

Ingredients:

- 2 cups mixed greens (spinach, arugula, and kale)
- ½ cup walnuts, roughly chopped
- ½ cup mixed berries (strawberries, blueberries, raspberries)
- ¼ cup feta cheese, crumbled

- Dressing: 3 tbsp extra virgin olive oil, 1 tbsp balsamicvinegar, salt, and pepper to taste

Preparation:

1. In a large salad bowl, combine mixed greens, walnuts, berries, andfeta cheese.
2. In a small bowl, whisk together olive oil, balsamic vinegar, salt, andpepper to make the dressing.
3. Drizzle the dressing over the salad and toss gently to combine.

How to Use: Enjoy this salad as a main dish or side to increase dietaryantioxidants for improved health and longevity.

Milk with Golden Turmeric

Intended Use: benefits from the anti-inflammatory and immune-boosting qualities of turmeric.

Ingredients:

- 1 cup almond milk or coconut milk
- 1 tsp turmeric powder
- ½ tsp cinnamon
- ¼ tsp ginger powder
- 1 tsp honey
- A pinch of black pepper

Preparation:

1. In a small saucepan, heat the milk gently and add turmeric,cinnamon, ginger, and black pepper.
2. Stir well and simmer for a few minutes without boiling.
3. Remove from heat and stir in honey.
4. Serve warm.

How to Use: Every day, especially before going to bed, have a cup of golden milk to boost your immune system and encourage its anti-inflammatory properties.

Herbal Anti-Aging Tea

Intended Use: combines a variety of anti-aging herbs to decrease inflammation and promote lifespan.

Ingredients:

- 1 tsp dried ginkgo biloba leaves
- 1 tsp dried green tea leaves
- ½ tsp dried turmeric
- ½ tsp dried ginger
- Honey or lemon to taste
- 2 cups boiling water

Preparation:

1. Combine ginkgo biloba, green tea, turmeric, and ginger in a teainfuser or teapot.
2. Pour boiling water over the herbs and let steep for 10 minutes.
3. Remove the infuser or strain the tea.
4. Add honey or lemon to taste.

Serve warm.

How to Use: Sip one to two cups every day to enhance lifespan, lower inflammation, and strengthen cognitive function.

Healthy Bone Broth

Intended Use: Rich in collagen, bone broth supports healthy intestinal flora, healthy joints, and general vigor.

Ingredients:

- 2 pounds mixed bones (beef, chicken, or fish)
- 2 carrots, chopped
- 2 celery stalks, chopped
- 1 onion, quartered
- 2 tbsp apple cider vinegar
- Water to cover
- Herbs and spices (optional: garlic, bay leaves, salt, pepper)

Preparation:

1. Place bones in a large pot and cover with water. Add apple cidervinegar; let sit

for 30 minutes.
2. Add vegetables and optional herbs/spices. Bring to a boil, thenreduce to a simmer.
3. Simmer for 12-24 hours, skimming foam and impurities from thesurface.
4. Strain the broth through a fine mesh strainer and store in therefrigerator or freezer.

How to Use: Consume 1 cup of bone broth daily, either on its own or as abase for soups and stews, to support digestive health and vitality.

Rich in Omega-3 Flaxseed Pudding

Intended Use: uses omega-3 fatty acids to lower inflammation and promote brain function.

Ingredients:

- ¼ cup flaxseeds, ground
- 1 cup almond milk
- 1 tsp vanilla extract
- 1 tbsp maple syrup
- Fresh berries for topping

Preparation:

1. In a bowl, mix ground flaxseeds with almond milk, vanilla extract,and maple syrup.
2. Refrigerate overnight or at least for 4 hours until it forms a pudding-like consistency.
3. Top with fresh berries before serving.

How to Use: Savor this pudding for breakfast or as a snack to increase your consumption of omega-3 fatty acids, which have anti-inflammatory and brain-healthy effects.

Balls of Spirulina Energy

Intended Use: uses nutrient-rich spirulina to promote detoxification and increase vitality.

Ingredients:

- 1 cup dates, pitted
- ½ cup almonds
- ½ cup cashews
- 2 tbsp spirulina powder
- 1 tbsp chia seeds

- Desiccated coconut for coating

Preparation:

1. In a food processor, blend dates, almonds, cashews, spirulina, andchia seeds until sticky.
2. Roll the mixture into small balls.
3. Coat each ball in desiccated coconut.
4. Refrigerate for at least an hour before serving.

How to Use: For a rapid energy boost and nutritional infusion, consume two to three energy balls as needed.

Digestive Aid Aloe Vera

Intended Use: Soothes the digestive tract and supports nutrient absorptionwith aloe vera.

Ingredients:

- ¼ cup pure aloe vera gel (ensure it's edible)
- 1 cup water or cucumber juice
- Juice of 1 lemon

Preparation:

1. Blend aloe vera gel with water or cucumber juice until smooth.
2. Stir in lemon juice.
3. Serve chilled for a refreshing and soothing drink.

How to Use: Consume half a cup in the morning on an empty stomach to assist healthy digestion and encourage internal restoration.

Kombucha for Digestive Health

Intended Use: increases immunity and enhances gut health with probiotic-rich kombucha.

Ingredients:

- 1 SCOBY (symbiotic culture of bacteria and yeast)
- 8 cups water
- ½ cup sugar

- 4 tea bags (green or black tea)
- 1 cup starter tea or vinegar

Preparation:

1. Boil water and dissolve sugar in it. Add tea bags and let steep untilthe water cools to room temperature.
2. Remove tea bags, add starter tea or vinegar, and transfer to a glassjar.
3. Gently add the SCOBY to the jar.
4. Cover with a cloth and secure with a rubber band. Ferment for 7-14days at room temperature.
5. Taste to check readiness. When satisfied, remove SCOBY and bottlethe kombucha.
6. Store bottled kombucha in the refrigerator.

How to Use: Consume 4–8 ounces of kombucha every day to promote general wellness and digestive health.

Avocado and Wild Salmon Salad

Intended Use: supplies proteins, antioxidants, and vital fatty acids for long-term heart function.

Ingredients:

- 2 cups mixed greens (spinach, arugula, lettuce)
- 1 avocado, sliced
- 4 ounces wild salmon, cooked and flaked
- ¼ red onion, thinly sliced
- Dressing: 2 tbsp olive oil, 1 tbsp lemon juice, salt, andpepper

Preparation:

1. Arrange mixed greens on a plate.
2. Top with avocado slices, salmon flakes, and red onion.
3. Whisk together olive oil, lemon juice, salt, and pepper to make thedressing.
4. Drizzle the dressing over the salad.

How to Use: Serve this salad as a nutritious lunch or dinner to supportcardiovascular health and contribute to a balanced, longevity-supporting diet.

IMMUNE SYSTEM MODULATION

Elderberry and Echinacea Immune Support Syrup

Intended Use: has antiviral and immune-boosting qualities throughout the cold and flu season.

Ingredients:

- ½ cup dried echinacea purpurea flowers or root
- ½ cup dried elderberries
- 4 cups water
- 1 cup raw honey

Preparation:

1. Combine echinacea and elderberries with water in a pot. Bring to aboil, then reduce heat and simmer for 45 minutes.
2. Strain the mixture through a fine mesh strainer, pressing to extract allliquid.
3. Allow the liquid to cool to lukewarm before stirring in honey.
4. Bottle the syrup and store in the refrigerator.

How to Use: Take 1 tbsp daily for immune support or every 3 hourswhen experiencing cold or flu symptoms.

Immune-Supporting Ferment of Garlic and Honey

Intended Use: combines the probiotic qualities of fermented honey with the antibacterial and antiviral effects of garlic to strengthen immune function.

Ingredients:

- 1 cup peeled garlic cloves
- Raw honey, enough to cover the garlic

Preparation:

1. Place garlic cloves in a clean jar.
2. Pour raw honey over the garlic until fully covered, leaving at least 1
3. inch of space at the top of the jar.
4. Cover the jar with a lid, allowing for some air exchange.

5. Let the jar sit at room temperature for 3-4 weeks, stirring or turningthe jar upside down daily.
6. Once fermented, store in the refrigerator.

How to Use: Eat one or two cloves of garlic every day, or take a tsp of honey to boost immunity.

Immune Tonic with Astragalus Root and Mushroom

Intended Use: uses medicinal mushrooms and astragalus root, both of which are recognized for their immune-boosting qualities, to strengthen and modify the immune system.

Ingredients:

- 1 tbsp dried astragalus root
- ½ cup mixed dried medicinal mushrooms (shiitake, reishi, maitake)
- 4 cups water
- 1 inch ginger, sliced
- Honey to taste

Preparation:

1. Combine astragalus root, medicinal mushrooms, and ginger in a largepot.
2. Add water and bring to a boil. Reduce heat and simmer for 1-2 hours,or until the liquid is reduced by half.
3. Strain the tonic and add honey to sweeten, if desired.
4. Store in a glass container in the refrigerator.

How to Use: To maintain the health of your immune system, drink half a cup of the tonic every day. Use during acute infections is not advised without first speaking with a healthcare professional.

Immune Tea with Thyme and Lemon Balm

Intended Use: uses antiviral and antibacterial herbs to support immune health while fostering calm and wellbeing.

Ingredients:

- 1 tsp dried lemon balm

- 1 tsp dried thyme
- 1 cup boiling water

Preparation:

1. Place lemon balm and thyme in a tea infuser or directly in a mug.
2. Pour boiling water over the herbs and cover.
3. Steep for 10 minutes, then strain.
4. Enjoy the tea warm, with honey if desired.

How to Use: To strengthen immunity, consume one or two cloves of garlic each day or take a tsp of honey.

Immune Ginger-Zinc Lozenges

Intended Use: uses the healing qualities of ginger and the immuno-stimulating effects of zinc to support immune function and relieve sore throats.

Ingredients:

- ½ cup fresh ginger, finely grated
- 2 cups water
- 1 cup raw honey
- ½ tsp zinc oxide powder (food grade)

Preparation:

1. Simmer ginger in water for 20 minutes to make a strong decoction.
2. Strain ginger, then add honey to the liquid and simmer untilthickened into a syrup.
3. Stir in zinc oxide powder until fully dissolved.
4. Pour the mixture into silicone molds and let set until firm.
5. Store in an airtight container.

How to Use: As required, dissolve one lozenge slowly in the mouth to boost the immune system and ease sore throats.

Beetroot and Carrot Immune-Boosting Juice

Intended Use: benefits immune system and blood health because to beetroot and carrot's high nutritional content.

Ingredients:

- 2 medium beetroots, peeled
- 4 large carrots, peeled
- 1 inch piece of ginger, peeled
- ½ lemon, peeled

Preparation:

1. Pass all ingredients through a juicer.
2. Stir the juice to combine flavors.
3. Serve immediately or store in the refrigerator for up to 24 hours.

How to Use: Drink 1 glass daily to support immune health and detoxificationprocesses.

Black pepper and turmeric for an immune-boosting shot

Intended Use: improves absorption with black pepper, boosts the immune system, and reduces inflammation with turmeric.

Ingredients:

- 1 tbsp turmeric powder
- A pinch of black pepper
- Juice of 1 lemon
- ½ cup water
- 1 tsp honey (optional)

Preparation:

1. Mix turmeric powder, black pepper, and lemon juice with water.
2. Stir in honey for sweetness if desired.
3. Drink immediately.

How to Use: Take one dose of this injection in the morning each day to help maintain a healthy immune system and lower inflammation.

Kefir Smoothie with Probiotics

Intended Use: Probiotic-rich kefir supports the regulation of the immune system and intestinal health.

Ingredients:

- 1 cup kefir

- ½ banana
- ½ cup mixed berries
- 1 tbsp flaxseed meal

Preparation:

1. Combine kefir, banana, berries, and flaxseed meal in a blender.
2. Blend until smooth.
3. Serve immediately for best taste and nutrient retention.

How to Use: Drink this smoothie as a snack or in the morning to help your immune system and digestive health.

Calm Licorice and Marshmallow Root Tea

Intended Use: uses licorice and marshmallow root to calm mucous membranes and modify the immunological response.

Ingredients:

- 1 tsp dried marshmallow root
- 1 tsp dried licorice root
- 1 cup boiling water

Preparation:

1. Combine marshmallow root and licorice root in a tea infuser or pot.
2. Pour boiling water over the herbs and steep for 10-15 minutes.
3. Strain and enjoy the tea warm.

How to Use: Drink 1-2 cups daily to support respiratory health and sootheirritated throats, particularly during cold and flu season.

Schisandra Berry Immune Tonic

Intended Use: increases immune function and resilience in general with adaptogenic schisandra berries.

Ingredients:

- 1 tbsp dried schisandra berries
- 2 cups water
- Honey to taste

Preparation:

1. Add schisandra berries to water in a small pot.
2. Bring to a boil, then reduce heat and simmer for 30 minutes.
3. Strain the tonic and add honey to sweeten if desired.
4. Allow cooling before drinking.

How to Use: Take one cup of tonic made from schisandra berries in the morning or afternoon to help your body's defenses against stress.

GET BETTER SLEEP

Tea with Chamomile and Lavender

Intended Use: The relaxing and sleep-inducing qualities of lavender and chamomile are well known.

Ingredients:

- 1 teaspoon dried lavender buds
- 1 tablespoon dried chamomile flowers
- Boiling water in two cups
- optional honey:

Preparation:

1. Fill a teapot or infuser with chamomile and lavender leaves.
2. Cover the herbs with boiling water and steep for five minutes.
3. Strain (if required) and add honey to taste, if preferred.

Toast with almond butter and bananas

Intended Use: Almond butter offers good fats, and bananas are high in potassium and magnesium. When combined, they facilitate rest and sleep.

Ingredients:

- One toasted slice of whole-grain bread
- One spoonful of butter made of almonds
- One banana, cut into slices

Preparation:

1. Toast should be topped with almond butter for preparation.
2. Slices of banana on top, then savor before going to bed.

Walnut and Kiwi Salad

Intended Use: Walnuts have melatonin, which helps induce sleep, and kiwis are rich in antioxidants and serotonin.

Ingredients:

- ¼ cup chopped walnuts
- Two peeled and sliced kiwis
- Honey is optional.

Preparation:

1. combine chopped walnuts and kiwi slices in a bowl.
2. If desired, drizzle with honey.

Warm Almond Milk Spiced with Cinnamon and Turmeric

Intended Use: Magnesium-rich almond milk, anti-inflammatory turmeric, and blood-sugar-stabilizing cinnamon all help promote sound sleep.

Ingredients:

- One cup almond milk
- One-half teaspoon of ground turmeric
- One-half teaspoon of ground cinnamon
- One tsp honey

Preparation:

1. In a small saucepan, warm the almond milk over medium heat.
2. Stir in honey, cinnamon, and turmeric.
3. Warm up, but do not boil, and then proceed to serve.

Pumpkin Seed Oatmeal with Cherries and Seeds

Intended Use: Rich in magnesium, cherries are one of the few food sources of melatonin, and oats are a healthy source of both complex carbohydrates and melatonin.

Ingredients:

- One cup milk or water
- One cup rolled oats
- One cup pumpkin seeds
- One cup dried cherries

Preparation:

1. Prepare oatmeal according to package directions, using milk or water.
2. Before serving, stir in the dried cherries and pumpkin seeds.

Blend of Herbal Tea for Sleeping

Intended Use: The intended use of this calming mixture of herbs is to promote rest and sleep.

Ingredients:

- One tsp of dehydrated valerian root
- One tsp of dried passionflower
- One tsp of dehydrated lemon balm
- Two cups of water that is boiling

Preparation:

1. In a teapot or infuser, mix herbs.
2. After adding boiling water to the herbs, let them steep for ten minutes.
3. After straining, sip a cup before going to bed.

Pineapple-infused cottage cheese

Intended Use: The slow-digesting casein protein included in cottage cheese helps to stave off hunger at night. Serotonin levels may be raised by pineapple.

Ingredients:

- Half a cup of cottage cheese
- ½ cup of pineapple dice

Preparation:

1. Just sprinkle chopped pineapple over cottage cheese and serve as a pre-bedtime snack.

Greek yogurt flavored with flaxseeds and honey

Intended Use: Flaxseeds contribute omega-3 fatty acids, while Greek yogurt supplies calcium, which aids in the brain's utilisation of tryptophan to make melatonin.

Ingredients:

- One cup of Greek yogurt
- One-third cup flaxseeds
- two tsp honey

Preparation:

1. Combining Greek yogurt with flaxseeds.
2. Drizzle with honey and
3. serve immediately.

Chamomile Lavender Tea

Intended Use: Calming and sleep-inducing qualities are well-known for chamomile and lavender.

Ingredients:

- One spoonful of dried flowers of chamomile
- One tsp of dried lavender buds
- Taste of honey
- One cup of water that is boiling

Preparation:

2. Put the lavender and chamomile flowers in a teapot or infuser.
3. Cover the herbs with boiling water, then let steep for five to ten minutes.
4. Before going to bed, strain (if needed) and add honey for sweetness.

Warm Milk with Turmeric

Intended Use: The compound curcumin, which is found in turmeric, may aid in promoting relaxation and lowering tension.

Ingredients:

- One cup of your preferred milk (cow, almond, etc.)
- One tsp powdered turmeric
- half a teaspoon of cinnamon
- One-fourth teaspoon of powdered ginger
- Taste-tested honey

Preparation:

1. In a small saucepan, warm the milk over low heat.
2. Add the ginger, cinnamon, and turmeric and stir.
3. After a few minutes of simmering, add honey to sweeten.
4. Warm up before retiring for the night.

Almond and Banana Smoothie

Intended Use: Magnesium and potassium, which are abundant in bananas, aid in the relaxation of muscles and nerves.

Ingredients:

- One ripe banana
- One spoonful of butter made of almonds
- One cup almond milk
- A small amount of nutmeg

Preparation:

1. Blend all ingredients until they are smooth.
2. For a calming effect, drink one hour before going to bed.

Avocado on Whole Grain Toast

Intended Use: While avocados supply magnesium, whole grains aid in raising tryptophan levels in the brain.

Ingredients:

- 1/2 ripe avocado and
- One slice of toasted whole grain bread
- To taste, add salt and pepper.

Preparation:

1. Mash the avocado and put it over the toast.
2. Add pepper and salt for seasoning.
3. Eat one to two hours before going to bed.

Tart Cherry Sauce with Cottage Cheese

Intended Use: Melatonin, which is present in tart cherries and the high casein protein content of cottage cheese, can both enhance the quality of your sleep.

Ingredients:

- Half a cup cottage cheese
- One-fourth cup of tart cherry juice
- One tsp honey
- A few frozen or fresh cherries

Preparation:

1. In small saucepan, warm honey and sour cherry juice. Simmer for a few minutes after adding the cherries.
2. Place the cottage cheese on top of the warm cherry sauce.
1. .

Walnut and Kiwi Salad

Intended Use: Walnuts are a good source of tryptophan, and kiwis are well-known for their serotonin levels.

Ingredients:

- Peel and cut into two ripe kiwis
- Several walnuts, coarsely chopped
- A honey drizzle

Preparation:

1. Mix walnuts and kiwi slices together in a bowl.
2. Before serving, pour some honey over it.

Lavender and Chamomile Sleeping Tea

Intended Use: helps the body unwind and gets ready for a good night's sleep thanks to the relaxing qualities of lavender and chamomile.

Ingredients:

- 1 tbsp dried chamomile flowers
- 1 tsp dried lavender flowers
- 1 cup boiling water
- Honey to taste (optional)

Preparation:

1. Combine chamomile and lavender in a tea infuser or directly in amug.
2. Pour boiling water over the herbs and cover.
3. Steep for 5-10 minutes, then remove the infuser or strain.
4. Sweeten with honey if desired.
5. Drink 30 minutes before bedtime.

How to Use: Consume this tea nightly as part of your bedtime routine toenhance sleep quality.

Herbal Tea for Sleeping

Intended Use: The intended use is as a calming blend of herbs that promote sleep.

Ingredients:

- One tsp of dehydrated valerian root
- One tsp of dehydrated lemon balm
- One tsp of dried passionflower
- One cup of water that is boiling

Preparation:

2. In a teapot or infuser, mix herbs.
3. After adding boiling water to the herbs, steep them for ten minutes.

Thirty minutes before bed, strain and sip

Banana Almond Smoothie Packed with Magnesium

Intended Use: Supports sleep by providing magnesium, known for itsmuscle-relaxing and nervous system-calming effects.

Ingredients:

- 1 ripe banana
- 1 cup almond milk
- 2 tbsp almond butter
- 1 tbsp chia seeds
- A pinch of cinnamon

Preparation:

1. Place all ingredients in a blender.
2. Blend until smooth.
3. Enjoy this smoothie 1-2 hours before bedtime.

How to Use: Enjoy this smoothie in the evening to take advantage of the magnesium found in chia seeds and almond butter, which helps to promote sound sleep.

Valerian Root Sleeping Tablets

Intended Use: uses valerian root, a powerful herbal sedative, to improve sleep quality and shorten the time it takes to fall asleep.

Ingredients:

- Valerian root powder
- Empty capsules

Preparation:

1. Fill empty capsules with valerian root powder using a capsule machine or a small spoon.
2. Store the filled capsules in a cool, dry place.

How to Use: 30 minutes before to going to bed, take one or two capsules. If more is required, start with the lesser dose and don't go beyond the suggested amount.

Warm Golden Milk for Slumber

Intended Use: uses the relaxing, anti-inflammatory properties of turmeric with the comforting warmth of milk to encourage sleep.

Ingredients:

- 1 cup milk (dairy or plant-based)
- ½ tsp turmeric powder
- ¼ tsp ginger powder
- A pinch of black pepper
- Honey to taste

Preparation:

1. Heat milk in a small saucepan over medium heat.

2. Stir in turmeric, ginger, and black pepper.
3. Simmer for a few minutes, then remove from heat.
4. Sweeten with honey.
5. Drink warm before going to bed.

How to Use: As part of your nightly ritual to help you fall asleep, have a cup of golden milk.

Calm Sleep Salve

Intended Use: uses a combination of essential oils that promote sleep to ease tension and quiet the mind in a calming salve.

Ingredients:

- ¼ cup coconut oil
- ¼ cup olive oil
- ¼ cup beeswax pellets
- 15 drops lavender essential oil
- 10 drops cedarwood essential oil
- Small jars or tins for storage

Preparation:

1. In a double boiler, melt coconut oil, olive oil, and beeswax together.
2. Remove from heat and let cool slightly.
3. Stir in lavender and cedarwood essential oils.
4. Pour into small jars or tins and let set until solid.

How to Use: Before going to bed, apply to the wrists, temples, and under the nose to promote calm and sleep.

Passionflower Sleep Tincture

Intended Use: Enhances the length and quality of sleep with passionflower, which has relaxing and sleep-inducing qualities.

Ingredients:

- ½ cup dried passionflower
- 1 cup vodka or apple cider vinegar
- Glass jar with lid

Preparation:

1. Place dried passionflower in the glass jar.
2. Cover with vodka or apple cider vinegar, ensuring herbs arecompletely submerged.
3. Seal the jar and store in a cool, dark place for 4-6 weeks, shakingevery few days.
4. Strain the tincture into a clean bottle.

How to Use: Half an hour before going to bed, take one or two droppers of the tincture under your tongue or in water.

Oatmeal and Lavender Bath Soak

Intended Use: A calming bath soak calms the body and gets the mind ready for sleep.

Ingredients:

- 1 cup Epsom salt
- ½ cup dried lavender flowers
- ½ cup ground oats
- Muslin bag or bath tea bag

Preparation:

1. Mix Epsom salt, lavender flowers, and ground oats together.
2. Fill a muslin bag or bath tea bag with the mixture.
3. Seal the bag tightly.
4. Place in a warm bath and soak for 20 minutes before bedtime.

How to Use: Use this bath soak as part of your nightly routine to relax thebody and mind, enhancing sleep quality.

Night Tea with Jujube Seeds

Intended Use: jujube seeds' inherent sedative qualities aid with sleep support.

Ingredients:

- 1 tbsp dried jujube seeds
- 1 cup boiling water

Preparation:

1. Crush jujube seeds slightly to release their active compounds.
2. Place seeds in a cup and cover with boiling water.

3. Cover and steep for 10 minutes.
4. Strain and drink the tea warm before bed.

How to Use: Drink jujube seed tea nightly to help ease into a restful sleep,particularly during periods of stress or insomnia.

Sleep-Improving Pillow Mist

Intended Use: uses essential oils to create a peaceful, tranquil environment that is ideal for sleeping in.

Ingredients:

- ½ cup distilled water
- 2 tbsp witch hazel or vodka
- 10 drops lavender essential oil
- 5 drops chamomile essential oil
- Spray bottle

Preparation:

1. Combine distilled water and witch hazel or vodka in a spray bottle.
2. Add lavender and chamomile essential oils.
3. Shake well to mix.
4. Spray lightly on pillows and bed linens before sleep.

How to Use: Use nightly to transform your bedroom into a calming oasis,promoting relaxation and deeper sleep.

Orange and Cedarwood Sleep Diffuser Mix

Intended Use: Fosters a restful sleep environment with the calming aroma ofcedarwood and uplifting scent of orange.

Ingredients:

- 5 drops cedarwood essential oil
- 5 drops orange essential oil
- Water for diffuser

Preparation:

1. Fill your diffuser with the recommended amount of water.

2. Add cedarwood and orange essential oils to the water.
3. Turn on the diffuser and let it run in your bedroom for 30 minutesbefore you go to sleep.

How to Use: Every night, use this diffuser combination to create a calm and relaxing environment in your bedroom that is favorable to sleep.

INCREASE GENERAL ENERGY

Maca Root Energy-Boosting Drink

Intended Use: Maca root, which is well-known for its adaptogenic and energy-boosting qualities, increases stamina and energy.

Ingredients:

- 1 tbsp maca powder
- 1 banana
- 1 cup spinach
- 1 tbsp almond butter
- 1 cup almond milk
- A handful of ice cubes

Preparation:

1. Place all ingredients in a blender.
2. Blend on high until smooth.
3. Serve immediately for the best taste and energy boost.

How to Use: For an energy boost, consume in the morning or right before working out.

Beetroot and Lemon Juice

Intended Use: boosts blood flow and stamina, giving off a natural energy boost.

Ingredients:

- 2 beetroots, peeled and chopped
- Juice of 1 lemon
- 1 inch ginger, peeled
- Water, as needed

Preparation:

1. Add all ingredients to a blender, adding enough water to blendsmoothly.
2. Strain the mixture to obtain a clear juice.
3. Serve the juice chilled or over ice.

How to Use: Have a glass in the morning or before working out to increase energy and endurance.

Bits of Spirulina Energy

Intended Use: has spirulina, a plant high in vitamins and minerals, which gives you a rapid and wholesome energy boost.

Ingredients:

- 1 cup dates, pitted
- ½ cup oats
- ¼ cup almond butter
- 2 tbsp spirulina powder
- Desiccated coconut for coating

Preparation:

1. In a food processor, blend dates, oats, almond butter, and spirulinauntil the mixture sticks together.
2. Roll the mixture into small balls.
3. Coat each ball with desiccated coconut.
4. Refrigerate for at least 30 minutes before serving.

How to Use: When you need a fast energy boost, eat one or two energy bits.

Herbal Tea with Ginseng

Intended Use: Stimulates physical and mental activity in individuals whofeel weak and tired with ginseng, a potent herbal stimulant.

Ingredients:

- 1 tsp dried ginseng root
- 1 cup boiling water

Preparation:

1. Place ginseng root in a cup.
2. Pour boiling water over the root and steep for 5-10 minutes.
3. Strain and drink the tea warm.

How to Use: To get over a midday slump, have one cup in the early afternoon or in the morning to boost your energy.

Drink with Chia Seed Hydration

Intended Use: Improves hydration and energy levels with chia seeds, knownfor their high omega-3 content and hydration properties.

Ingredients:

- 2 tbsp chia seeds
- 2 cups coconut water
- Juice of 1 lime
- Honey to taste

Preparation:

1. In a jar, mix chia seeds with coconut water.
2. Let sit for 20 minutes until the chia seeds have swollen.
3. Add lime juice and honey to taste. Stir well.
4. Serve chilled.

How to Use: Drink before working out in the morning to keep hydrated and alert.

Green Tea and Mint Refresher

Intended Use: Benefits from the stimulating properties of green tea and mint, which also raise energy and mental alertness.

Ingredients:

- 1 green tea bag or 1 tsp loose green tea leaves
- 5 fresh mint leaves
- Honey to taste
- 1 cup hot water

Preparation:

1. Steep green tea and mint leaves in hot water for 3-5 minutes.
2. Remove the tea bag or strain the leaves.
3. Add honey to taste and stir well.
4. Serve warm or chilled with ice.

How to Use: Enjoy a cup in the morning or during a mid-afternoon break torefresh and energize.

Milk of Ashwagandha

Intended Use: uses ashwagandha, an adaptogen that aids in stress management, to lower tension and boost energy.

Ingredients:

- 1 tsp ashwagandha powder
- 1 cup milk (dairy or plant-based)
- Honey or maple syrup to taste
- A pinch of cinnamon (optional)

Preparation:

1. Warm the milk in a saucepan over low heat.
2. Add ashwagandha powder and cinnamon, if using. Stir well.
3. Remove from heat before it boils and sweeten with honey or maplesyrup.
4. Serve warm.

How to Use: To unwind and get ready for a restful sleep, sip on a cup of ashwagandha milk in the evening. This will help to support your energy levels the following day in an indirect way.

Almond and Quinoa Energy Bars

Intended Use: provides a long-lasting energy boost from the protein-rich quinoa and the good fats found in almonds.

Ingredients:

- 1 cup cooked quinoa
- ½ cup almonds, chopped
- ¼ cup honey
- ¼ cup peanut butter
- ½ tsp vanilla extract
- A pinch of salt

Preparation:

1. Preheat the oven to 350°F (175°C).

2. In a bowl, mix all ingredients until well combined.
3. Press the mixture into a lined baking tray.
4. Bake for 20 minutes, or until golden.
5. Let cool and cut into bars.

How to Use: To keep your energy levels up throughout the day, eat an energy bar as a snack in between meals.

Herbal Energy Concoction

Intended Use: Boosts energy and vitality with a blend of energizing herbs.

Ingredients:

- 1 part ginseng root
- 1 part eleuthero root
- 1 part green tea leaves
- Vodka or apple cider vinegar for extraction

Preparation:

1. Combine herbs in a jar.
2. Cover with vodka or apple cider vinegar, ensuring herbs are fully submerged.
3. Seal the jar and store in a dark place for 4-6 weeks, shaking daily.
4. Strain the tincture into a clean bottle.

How to Use: Take 1-2 droppers of the tincture in water or directly under the tongue in the morning or early afternoon for an energy boost.

Rose Rhodiola capsules

Intended Use: Rhodiola rosea, which is well-known for its adaptogenic and energetic qualities, increases both mental and physical stamina.

Ingredients:

- Rhodiola rosea powder
- Empty capsules

Preparation:

1. Fill empty capsules with Rhodiola rosea powder using a capsulefilling machine or manually with a small spoon.

2. Store the capsules in a cool, dry place.

How to Use: Take one capsule in the morning or early afternoon, especiallyduring periods of increased stress or when additional energy is needed.

Avocado with Green Tea Smoothie

Intended Use: This smoothie provides a steady burst of energy by combining the natural caffeine found in green tea with the beneficial fats found in avocado.

Ingredients:

- One cup of chilled brewed green tea
- One mature avocado
- half a cup of spinach
- One tablespoon honey (optional)
- a few cubes of ice

Preparation:

1. Put everything into a blender.
2. Process until smooth on high speed blending.
3. Serve right away for a hit of revitalization.

How to Use: Have a drink in the afternoon to get out of the slump or in the morning to get your day going.

Pudding with Chia Seeds

Intended Use: Chia seeds are high in protein, fiber, and omega-3 fatty acids, this pudding is a great way to boost energy for breakfast or a snack.

Ingredients:

- Three tablespoons of chia seeds
- One cup coconut milk
- One tablespoon of maple syrup
- Half a teaspoon vanilla extract
- Topping: fresh berries

Preparation:

1. In a bowl, combine chia seeds, coconut milk, maple syrup, and vanilla.

2. Store in the fridge for at least 4 hours or overnight.
3. Before serving, give it a good stir and add some fresh berries on top.

How to Use: Savor this for breakfast or as a snack for a sustained energy source.

Smoothie with Berries and Beets

Intended Use: Berries contribute antioxidants, and beetroots' high nitrate content enhances blood flow and boosts energy.

Ingredients:

- One little beetroot, sliced and peeled
- 1/2 cup of mixed berries, either frozen or fresh
- One banana
- one cup coconut water or water
- a few cubes of ice

Preparation:

1. Put everything into a blender.
2. Process until smooth on high speed blending.
3. Serve right away and experience its invigorating properties.

How to Use: Perfect to have in the morning or right before working out.

Revitalizing Verdant Juice

Intended Use: This juice, which is high in vitamins and minerals from green veggies, is meant to provide you energy throughout the day without the need of caffeine.

Ingredients:

- Two cups of spinach
- One cucumber
- One green apple
- Quarter of a lemon, peeled
- One-inch ginger root

Preparation:

1. Use a juicer to extract the components.
2. For optimal absorption and an energy boost, drink right away on an empty stomach.

Quinoa Breakfast Bowl Packed with Protein

Intended Use: Quinoa is a complete protein that provides all nine essential amino acids, which makes this dish a potent source of energy.

Ingredients:

- Half a cup of cooked quinoa
- One-fourth cup almond milk
- 1 tablespoon almond butter
- One banana, cut into slices
- A sprinkling of cinnamon
- A little handful of almonds or walnuts

Preparation:

1. Over low heat, reheat the cooked quinoa with almond milk.
2. Mix thoroughly after adding the almond butter.
3. Spoon into a bowl and garnish with nuts, cinnamon, and sliced bananas.

How to Use: Perfect for a hearty and stimulating breakfast.

Citrus and Spinach Salad

Intended Use: Packed with iron and vitamin C, this salad promotes better iron absorption and raises energy levels.

Ingredients:

- Two cups of raw spinach
- One peeled and segmented orange
- Slicing 1/4 cup of almonds
- Two tablespoons of olive oil
- One tablespoon balsamic vinegar
- To taste, add salt and pepper.

Preparation:

1. In a salad bowl, mix spinach, orange segments, and almonds.
2. Combine olive oil, balsamic vinegar, salt, and pepper in a whisk.
3. Pour the dressing over the salad and give it a little stir.

How to Use: Serve as a light lunch or as an accompaniment.

Ginger tea and turmeric

Intended Use: Due to their anti-inflammatory qualities, ginger and turmeric can increase energy levels by easing weariness and enhancing digestion.

Ingredients:

- 1 teaspoon ground turmeric
- Half a teaspoon of powdered ginger, or a tiny piece of fresh ginger
- One cup of heated water
- Taste of honey
- A spritz of lemon juice

Preparation:

1. Stir thoroughly after adding ginger and turmeric to boiling water.
2. Give it five to ten minutes to steep.
3. If using fresh ginger, strain; otherwise, taste and add honey and lemon juice.

How to Use: Use in the morning or anytime you feel like you need a pick-me-up.

Smoothie with Avocado and Spinach

Intended Use: The iron in spinach and the healthy fats in avocados help to maintain energy levels throughout the day.

Ingredients:

- One ripe avocado, ½
- One cup of raw spinach
- One banana
- One cup of coconut water
- One spoonful of chia seeds
- Cubes of ice

Preparation:

1. Combine together all of the ingredients in a blender.
2. Process till smooth.
3. Enjoy cold, ideally first thing in the morning or prior to exertion.

Pudding with Chia Seeds

Intended Use: Packed with fiber and omega-3 fatty acids, chia seeds are an ideal slow-release energy snack or breakfast.

Ingredients:

- Three tsp of chia seeds
- 1 cup almond milk without sugar
- One spoonful of maple syrup
- One-half teaspoon of vanilla extract
- Topping: fresh berries

Preparation:

1. Combine almond milk, vanilla, maple syrup, and chia seeds in a basin.
2. Store in the fridge all night.
3. Top with fresh berries and serve.

Breakfast Bowl with Quinoa

Intended Use: Quinoa is an excellent source of complex carbs and a complete protein that provides sustained energy.

Ingredients:

- One cup of cooked quinoa
- One-third tsp flaxseed meal
- ½ chopped apple and ¼ cup chopped walnuts
- To taste, cinnamon
- One cup almond milk

Preparation:

1. Reheat the cooked quinoa.
2. Add the chopped apple, walnuts, and flaxseed meal and stir.
3. Add almond milk and cinnamon.
4. Warm up and serve.

GET YOUR BONUS HERE:

Made in the USA
Las Vegas, NV
21 April 2024